D0728951

Here's what reviewers are saying about *Coming Home:*

It is beautifully written, extremely helpful. I am proud of Deborah's work.
—Elizabeth Kubler-Ross

...teaches an important lesson to those of us who must confront the death of a loved one.
—The Los Angeles Times

A wide ranging discussion about caring at home for a terminally ill patient...covers such practical matters as arranging for homemaker services, obtaining financial aid and administering medications.
—Changing Times Magazine

...a pioneering work. As a comprehensive resource book it is invaluable for family and friends wishing to help an individual die at home...It is a welcome guide.
—Open Hands Quarterly

...a complete and well-researched reference dealing very practically with the whole range of physical, emotional and spiritual problems in this complex situation.
—New Life News

Coming Home

A Guide To Home Care
For The Terminally Ill

The medical, health and supportive procedures in this book are based on the training, personal experiences and research of the author and on recommendations of responsible medical and nursing sources. But because each person and situation is unique, author and publisher urge the reader to check with a qualified health professional before using any procedure where there is any question as to its appropriateness.

The publisher does not advocate the use of any particular healing technique or practice but believes the information presented in this book should be available to the public.

Because some risks may be involved, the author and publisher assume no responsibility for any adverse effects or consequences resulting from the use of any of the suggestions, preparations or procedures in this book. Please do not use the book if you are unwilling to assume those risks. Feel free to consult a physician or other qualified health professional. It is a sign of wisdom, not timidity or cowardice, to seek a second or third opinion.

This book may be quoted up to one full page without written permission, provided credit is given including the name of this book, the author, and John Muir Publications.

Cover by Michaellallen McGuire
Illustrated by Extension Seven

Published by John Muir Publications, Inc.
P.O. Box 613
Santa Fe, New Mexico 87504

Library of Congress Catalogue Card No. 84-61564
ISBN 0-912528-39-7

Book trade distributor   W.W. Norton & Co., Inc.
500 Fifth Avenue
New York, NY 10036

To Mom and Dad, Judy and Suzy, Auntie Thelma,
Ben and Joshua
for giving me so much love that I could
look at things I was afraid of.

ACKNOWLEDGEMENTS

I give again the thanks I've already given many times in my heart to John Muir, Mary Conley, Dad and all the others who shared with me the incredible gift of their dyings and deaths. And to all the families and friends with the courage to make their dying at home possible, particularly my Mom, Craig Conley and Jean Pallares, and Eve Muir. Thank you, dear Eve, for also caring enough about the book to spend so much time helping me make my vision understandable to others.

Each person who helped with the book cared in his or her own way that there be less fear in the world and a greater acceptance of life including death. The caring of each increased the light in the world. A loving thanks to each friend, advisor, supporter, teacher and inspirer along the way: Ken and Barbara Luboff, Paul Abrams, Richard Polese and all the John Muir Publications staff, Leigh Peacocke, Gathanna Parmenas, Carolyn Silver, Robert Waterman, Malka Eisgrau, Sally Kingsmill, Angie Dickson, Jay and Mary Lou Ridinger, Susan Rush, Anna Roy, Forest Smith, Henry Weinhofen, Angela Werneke, Jim Exten, Glen Strock, Zoey Viles, Margaret and Bob Chisolm, Tom McCann, Elisabeth Kübler-Ross, Mother Teresa and my own inner guides.

Contents

Chapter 4:
GETTING ON WITH IT:
PREPARATIONS AND HOMECOMING   89

Chapter 5:
MEDICAL CONSIDERATIONS   96

In the Beginning there was Life. And Life seemed to be without form. It was indistinguishable. So Death was created to give form to Life. And then people began to become attached to Life and see Death as the enemy. In some places people saw Life as the enemy, the place of suffering, and Death, the friend.

And now we come to a place where we see that both are One.

So those of us who made an enemy of Death, must make of Death a friend. And those who made an enemy of Life, must make of Life a friend.

Introduction

Ten years ago I was wandering around the world looking outside myself for some teacher or teaching to help me understand what my life was all about. I decided to return to the clarity I remembered in a small village at the foot of Mount Machupuchere, in Nepal.

In Pokkara, I found a Sherpa guide who volunteered to act as interpreter and go with me to the village to find a house. The next day two Tibetan women carried my bags up the mountain trails to the tiny mud house we had found and I set up housekeeping. I quit trying to figure "it" all out and just lived contentedly with the villagers, taking photographs and recording the sounds and music of village life.

After a few weeks I began to have nightmares: I or someone in my family was dying. Each day I was afraid of what the next night might bring. One day a few months later a Sherpa stopped by with a valentine from Mom and Dad and a copy of *Newsweek* magazine with Mother Teresa's picture on the cover. That night I dreamed about her. The next morning I decided the only way to overcome my fear of death was to put myself in the middle of it. I would go to Calcutta and ask Mother Teresa if I could work in a *Hydray House*, one of the homes she created for people dying on the streets. *Hydray* is Sanscrit for "heart."

By the time I arrived in Calcutta, I was so sick with dysentery and worms that getting out of bed to call Mother Teresa was a great effort. When I did, I found her easy to talk with. I told her about my dreams and asked if I could see her. Very lovingly she said, "Come right over, my child." I dragged myself to the main convent in Calcutta and asked her my crucial question, "Can I work for a few months in one of your homes for the dying?" She answered, "No, my child. Go home. There is sadness and suffering right around you at home." Then, feeling desperate and lonely, I asked, "Can I adopt a child from the orphanage?" Again she answered, "No, my child. Go home and work with the sadness and loneliness around you." And I did—first with the fear, sadness and loneliness in myself. And the key has been *hydray,* the heart—transforming the fear that keeps hearts closed.

I began writing this book after two friends I love very much were cared for at home until they died. Then I worked with terminally ill patients and their families at our local hospital and with some who chose to die at home. While I was doing the final editing on this book, my father died at home.

Before the deaths of my two friends, when I thought of dying I felt stupid, which made me afraid or angry—so I pretended indifference. As a teenager, a gray squirrel on a country road was the only living thing I'd seen die. I shuddered as I watched its death dance in the rearview mirror. A public road! It's out of place, out of the natural. Everyone knows animals go away to die in hidden places. For three days I kept off the road while trying to figure out where this death fit into the scheme of things. Later in life I shot a few deer, and blanked that out. I saw my grandfather dead but didn't see how he got that way.

Not until past thirty did I really become aware that people were dying around me all the time; that *I* was dying all the time, parts of me, old cells, old ideas, old ways of being. Death was hidden out of sight in hospitals, in statistics, in a compartment of my being I didn't look at. I saw a friend lonely and isolated because fear kept friends from talking with her about the most important thing happening in her life—her dying.

Then I was angry, truly angry—anger born from awareness of my own ignorance and fear. I felt cheated. Most of us are cheated out of the fullness of life by fear and embarass-ment. We experience the pain and joy of birth and life and then many of us deny ourselves our death, the closure of a circle. Denial comes from fear... our fear, doctors' fear, loved ones' fear, our whole culture's fear.

As I began to accept dying and death as part of my experience of life, my anger was transformed into compassion, my fear into love.

This book has grown from a greater sense of wholeness (holiness) that has come from working with dying people and the deaths and rebirths within myself. It covers the practical information needed to help alleviate many of our fears. "Practical" includes not only the "what-to-do and how-to-do-it" of physical care, but also mental, emotional and spiritual support. Once the needs for comfort and relief from pain are met, spiritual food can be more nourishing than a glass of carrot juice or a hamburger. Supporting a home-dying is a wonderful opportunity to learn that spiritual support can be practical and physical care can be spiritual.

The book, then, is a synthesis of my psychological and spiritual understandings and the basic information on physical care needed to support someone who lives at home until he or she dies. It includes things to keep in mind when making the decision where to die. And, if home is the choice, what to do about family morale, pacing yourself, pain relief, calling a doctor, giving injections and enemas, taking care of your feelings, etc. Although the book is directed principally to the family and friends, much of it can be shared with the dying person as well.

I share with you my reality, my vision at this time in my life. Your reality, including your spiritual understanding and approach to death may be different. Use this book as a tool to help find the answers in yourself. If I use words that are not your words, let us move deeper than the word level... to the heart.

Trust yourself! We learn by having the courage to enter another's reality without seeing it as a threat and we can do this only if we trust ourselves. Sometimes seeing ideas in print convinces us that someone "out there" is *the expert* who knows more than we do about our experience. Anyone outside of ourselves can only be a provider of information or inspiration. You're the only expert on your reality. The appropriate way to work with dying is the way the dying person and you choose. And if some of your choices are different from theirs, you can do it your way when it's your turn.

Dying is the process of the life forces withdrawing from the body and death the moment of withdrawal. We often hear that life and death are opposites. To me, the opposites are birth and death. One describes entering into form, the other leaving form. Which is which depends on your perspective. Either way, life continues without end. So in this book "dying," "death," "dead," and "died" refer only to change in form and do not mean "the end," "the final disaster," or the "uncontrollable enemy." I see death as a friend on our way home to more life.

I believe at some level of our being we decide when we're going to die. After that our only choices are our attitude about dying and, sometimes, where it will take place. Both affect the quality of the time we have, and the latter may affect the quantity.

Accepting death is a process of surrender, of letting go and accepting life as it is rather than how we think it should be. Exquisite beauty and meaning can be present in dying when we and the dying person accept in our hearts that life is following its natural course, and when we cooperate with life instead of fighting against it. When we do, we no longer feel separate from each other and from life; we see the underlying unity of everything.

Love makes being alive worthwhile. Love transforms fear. Caring for a dying person is an opportunity to increase our capacity to love by decreasing fear. Within each of us is love, a lover, and a beloved—so we can't really lack love, someone to love, or someone to love us. But fear keeps hearts closed, which prevents us from experiencing this. Fear prevents surrendering and makes us feel separate and alone.

Fear projects awful things that may happen, especially while someone is dying. I've never encountered anything awful in all the home dyings I've been involved with. And before I worked with dying people I seemed to be the ideal candidate for *not* being able to handle dying. I had a long history of passing out in health class, at the sight of blood, or just visiting a friend in the hospital; I was terrified each time I got a shot, and, on more than one occasion, threw up when someone near me did.

To be afraid of death is to be afraid of life. The book is about acknowledging our fears, while at the same time moving through them toward greater love, joy and freedom as we experience dying.

One way our culture teaches fear of death (life) is by making security a goal. Total security is, of course, an illusion. Life is a process of change and inherent in change are vulnerability and risk. At any moment our plans for the future can disintegrate. Holding on to security or chasing after it creates more insecurity and fear. And do we really want it anyway? Maximum security is prison, not life.

We break the circle of fear and insecurity when we live each moment as it comes. You can do this right now with this "dying" you're living.

Peace is possible in this moment. It's not out there somewhere in the future. The future never really comes, anyway. By the time it gets to us, it's the present.

Focusing on life as a process instead of a goal has helped me accept death. I accept that at any point in time a process is complete. So at each moment each of us is complete and whole. No one dies before the purpose of his or her life is fulfilled even if we cannot understand that purpose. I believe that a child who dies young or someone who dies unexpectedly dies complete. Perhaps some of their projects aren't complete but who we are is not our unfinished work, projects or goals. The purpose of goals is just to give us a sense of direction. When life is seen as a process and not a goal, death loses much of its sting and,

> *Today is a good day to die for all the things of my life are here.* —Crazy Horse

Like living, dying has its share of sadness and joy. The sadness of letting go of a person we love is tempered if we remember to hold everyone lightly, knowing they are "just on loan." When someone we love is dying, we tend to focus on sadness, not on joy. But it's a choice. We can allow joy into this often most painful experience of our lives; the quiet joy of sharing love and caring, of seeing a loved one content, of touching into timelessness.

If we live each moment of each day fully, we transcend time. Each moment then becomes an eternity and we have all the time in the universe to share with this dying person we love. It doesn't matter how long we live, only *how* we live the time we have. It's possible to create of this experience a beautiful time in your life.

The increased love and compassion we can learn while caring for someone who dies at home will help us through our initial loneliness. If the death has not been sudden, there's been time between smoothing sheets, emptying bedpans, holding hands and talking of what may come, for grieving and resolving any unclarity with the dying person. There's been time to begin a gradual adjustment to earthly life without this person.

Because dying is living intensified, the qualities most needed to support someone dying are the same ones needed for living fully: love, compassion, courage, serenity, humor, humility and right use of will—allowing others to live or die as they choose as long as they take responsibility for their choices.

By taking responsibility for dying, we reclaim responsibility for living and regain lost personal power. One way to take responsibility is to stop playing victim to our culture's pressure to go away quietly and die in the sterility of a nursing home or hospital. Who wants to be seen as a forthcoming vacancy! We can die *right here* amidst the people and things we love, the kids, the dog, the garden, our favorite chair.

As you live this dying, be gentle with yourself and love yourself. There's no need to judge or blame yourself or feel guilty. Our lives are a learning process in which we outgrow some old thoughts and feelings as we increase in wisdom. Blame or guilt about the past is punishing ourselves for learning! Keep forgiving yourself for being so hard on yourself, and remember that what we're accustomed to calling "mistakes" are really experiences to learn from.

In this book I use the phrases "dying person," "sick person" and "patient" to save more convoluted wording. Inherent in these phrases are notions that hold us to old patterns. *We're all dying.* I don't believe there is such a thing as a "sick person"—only people with imbalances between their bodies, minds, feelings and souls. "Patient" has an impersonal quality which denies our uniqueness and humanness and promotes the illusion that a dying person's experience is separate from ours. Our experiences aren't separate. *We* aren't separate.

Chapter I

Three Experiences with Dying at Home

I'd like to share with you my first two experiences with friends who died at home and my dad's death. Perhaps after reading about them, dying at home won't seem like walking into the unknown. At least their stories may give you an idea of what it can be like. Their deaths and each home death I have been privileged to share was unique. And each was a song of love.

John

John Muir was best known for his book, *How to Keep Your Volkswagen Alive, A Manual of Step-by-Step Procedures for the Compleat Idiot.* To his friends he is remembered for his love, generosity and heckling to remind us to live in the *present.*

I met John and his wife and partner, Eve, nine years ago in a colonial town in the mountains of Mexico. The big treat in San Miguel was to go to John and Eve's on Thursday afternoons to soak in the hot pool and talk about our projects and dreams. John had a special gift for sharing love and financial support to help make his friends' dreams come true without undermining their own dignity or initiative.

Over a number of years, a loving family of friends grew that supported each of us in being and doing whatever we chose. Some wanted and needed John to be the patriarch and John allowed it. He was a delightful patriarch... enjoying the love given him and having fun with the power. At the same time, he encouraged us to take responsibility for ourselves and believed "humans have evolved to where leaders are no longer necessary."

If a 'hero' is a person who is true to his or her beliefs and inspires others, John was a hero. Physically he looked the part. He was a huge, lion-like, tawny-colored being with blue eyes that *saw* what they were looking at. He did what he wanted to do and thought what he wanted to think... which was often very unorthodox. Without regard to the traditional value of job security, at various times he was musician, sailor, mechanic, welder, structural engineer, builder, and author; also beatnik, hippie, philosopher, lover, husband, and father. He traveled the U.S. and Mexico in a converted 33-passenger army bus and sailed a Chinese junk until it sank in a hurricane off Cape Hatteras.

When no publisher wanted the "Volkswagen Idiot Book," John and Eve had enough faith in it to sell a house and start their own publishing company. They made a reasonable fortune and shared it. Each January, John held a month-long business meeting/party at the beach in Mexico and paid for friends who otherwise could not have come to share their ideas and manuscripts.

John was unusual in his incessant curiosity about life. His second book, *The Velvet Monkey Wrench,* was his blueprint for a society based on agreement among people to respect each other and the land. John and I became closer amidst yelling, steaming and thoughtful explanations while I helped to edit it. Later, after John, Eve, another friend and I trekked through Nepal, John continued to work on a book about the Life Force, the energy that gives life to matter. At different times he called this proposed book "The Doctrine of Admitt-ance," "Choices," "Sharing," or "Taking Responsibility for Ourselves So Leaders Are No Longer Necessary."

John loved and was fascinated by women. There were generally lots around. He felt they held a clue for him about the Life Force. He *knew* it was connected to the balance of male and female energy in the universe. In his last couple of years, John seemed almost controlled by his search to under-stand it. A number of friends asked him to let go of the book for a while because it seemed to be making him sick. John would not let go.

One hot June morning in Oregon, he stood up after his usual three-minute headstand and fell from dizziness. The dizziness continued and couldn't be diagnosed—a CAT Scan showed nothing, his ears and eyes were perfect. He asked Eve, seemingly out of the blue, "Is this just an incon-venience or is this death?"

By late August the dizziness was worse and his writing shaky. A second CAT Scan showed a growth on his brain. He decided to have the tumor removed to see whether or not it was malignant. The operation verified a fast-growing malig-nant tumor, an offshoot from one in his lung. The doctors said, "Two months to two years." At that time John was 59.

He recovered quickly from the operation and refused radiation therapy, saying, "If I'm wrong will you dance on my grave?" Then he and Eve drove to San Francisco to get more information about possible treatments and to find laetrile . . . a clandestine search. Armed with laetrile, they headed to New Mexico, camping leisurely in their VW van in places that were magic for them, like the red and white sandstone forma-tions of southern Utah.

In Santa Fe John returned to the acupuncturist who had told him before the dizziness started, "You're in a very dangerous position." John had interpreted this to mean his cholesterol level and blood pressure were too high. He tried acupuncture again but this time it was too painful. Except for occasional forays into ice cream, he stuck to a vegetable diet—quite a change for a "meat and potatoes man." He denied he had cancer and told us not to mention his condition. Every morning he dictated his life force ideas into a tape recorder.

One day in mid-October John woke up with a terrific headache. Pressure from the growing tumor was causing fluid to collect in his head. He agreed to have the fluid drained. Although this was supposed to be a relatively simple procedure, it impaired his speech. This was a kind of death for John. He loved to talk and was frustrated about losing control and slurring his words. His thinking remained clear, however.

The doctors said if he stayed in the hospital he would be hooked up to life support systems. After a radiantly loving session playing guitar and singing around his hospital bed, it was obvious that his friends were too many and too noisy for a hospital. He wanted out and we wanted him out. Elizabeth, his friend and former wife and mother of their son Star, spoke everyone's feeling, "The quality of life is more important than the quantity."

John and Eve didn't have their own home in Santa Fe, so a friend loaned them a large, empty adobe. In the four hours before the ambulance arrived with John, we made the house a home . . . rugs, pillows, wall hangings, rented TV and hospital bed, a complete kitchen, and a schedule for cooking and sitting with John in two-hour shifts. No one in particular directed. Each person sensed the needs and went about fulfilling them.

It was one of those specially glorious Autumn afternoons in the mountains when the ambulance pulled up. John was carried on a stretcher through the wooden gate and down the stone garden path. The sun shone on him through golden aspen leaves. After we tucked him in bed next to a window partially opened to the fresh mountain air, he seemed relieved and content. Some of us fussed with food; others gathered around the fireplace and played guitars. Often someone tiptoed in to see John sleeping, not because he needed checking, just for the joy of seeing him at *home*. That evening friends were called all over the country. "If you need to say goodbye to John in person, it's time to come." Already 15 to 20 of us had gathered, eight lived or camped around the house.

John orchestrated his dying as he did his living. Rusty, a nurse and masseur friend from Mexico, became the coordinator for his needs. Some of the family still had ideas about saving his body and the first morning home John said, "Let the kids test their theories." He believed actions are things to learn from. There are no mistakes, no being wrong. If we do nothing, we learn nothing.

In fairness to the different treatments that were tried—diet, laetrile, poultices, acupuncture, etc.—I feel they were tested after John had already decided at some level to die.

My personal concern was his preparation for the soul voyage rather than the attempts to save the body. I gave him Bach Flowers, tinctures of flower essences that work on an energetic principle which many believe help integrate the personality and the soul (see Appendix B).

Day by day I watched John and Eve as they decided what he did and did not want. He continued to take laetrile and although he was very uncomfortable he did not have severe pain. The laetrile and Bach Flowers seemed to have positive benefits in terms of pain control, although it's hard to say because doctors estimate that up to 50 percent of terminal cancer patients don't have pain.

Within the family, loving factions developed over diet. Was it best to maintain an extreme cleansing diet or was it too late? John wanted ice cream, not wheatgrass juice and raw vegetables. Seemed reasonable to me. Ice cream and cigarettes were sneaked to him to protect the feelings of friends not ready for him to let go of his body.

Time seemed to stand still as we shared those last few weeks together. When we weren't massaging, bathing, feeding or just being with him, we sat around the fire, reminisced about shared experiences, and caught up on the latest details in our lives. In the evenings some made a circle of power for healing around him, some chanted. An Indian medicine man was called and made a "helping the spirit to leave ceremony." Another minister from the Native American Church, who performed John and Eve's wedding ceremony ten years earlier, came to give his blessings. An oncologist, two unconventional MDs, and a homeopath with whom John had long evening visits, were in and out.

Having friends to share this dying experience was very supportive, though not all roses. Two couples who'd fought and weren't speaking, gracefully, and I imagine with difficulty, laid aside their grievances. Quarrels seemed less important in the face of dying. One night a friend of John and Eve's brought her drunk and suicidal brother to the house and left him there while she went out dancing. I was outraged. How could anyone be so thoughtless? John was dying in the next room! Eve found it perfectly OK and without words she helped me understand that there was enough love for everyone. It was an important lesson for me about operating out of plenty instead of scarcity. But it still took me a while to let go of my anger. Several of us had opportunities to examine jealousy or irritation as we imagined that so-and-so was 'more important' or 'taking over.' And all this was OK and part of the learning.

Then there was the afternoon two friends put a clay poultice on the back of John's neck and left him to go play with a video camera in the living room. Everyone was making so much noise that no one heard John's bellow for help until after the poultice burned him. He was furious and hollered, "I want to see *ALL* of you with one of these on."

We all wondered what the family would be like without John. We wondered why he was dying when he seemed to live with such joy and enthusiasm. Some of our theories about his death told more about our relationship with him and what we were dealing with in our own lives than about the actual reasons for his death. I believe John and I had the same "dis-ease"—an attachment to being in control and resistance to surrendering. We were both stubborn and were both looking for answers outside of ourselves.

I now feel John's dying was his ultimate lesson in surrender. Without surrender, the feminine principle, he couldn't complete his ideas on the life force. If we haven't learned it before, dying can teach us surrender. And when we surrender, we open to the life force which is always within us. I sense that John wanted the answer to his question so much he created his dying to get the answer. It's been nearly as tough for me to let go of fantasies about the patriarch as it was for the patriarch to let go.

After it appeared obvious to us that there was no way to save his body, John seemed to be deciding whether to fight or to surrender to death. Some of us were reading Elisabeth Kübler-Ross's description of the stages of dying—denial and isolation, anger, bargaining, depression, and acceptance. I watched him go back and forth among them all.

Most of the time John denied he was dying; this left him in control but unable to find ways to heal himself. He bargained, "Let me just finish the book" or "Oh, OK, if Eve and I can just take a trip to Hawaii first." Off and on he was depressed. He said, "I was always afraid of being hurt and now I hurt." It was difficult to talk with John about dying because he hadn't accepted what was happening to him. He'd often said, "Death is the greatest adventure of them all. I'll see what it's like when I get there." Yet being angry and fighting seemed to clear the air so he could finally accept *his* dying. Once he did, it took him only a day and a half to die.

Still vivid images from those weeks are Eve's graceful calm and humour; the oncologist in suit and tie and the medicine man in a black feathered hat crossing paths in John's room—and John chuckling; Eve lifting cupped hands of new fallen snow to John so he could enjoy the first snowfall; the two of them cuddled in the narrow hospital bed; Eve and Elizabeth (John's former wife) working side by side bathing him; John and I watching Walter Cronkite report the news while Eve was off dancing; his telling everyone who brought up business, "Look, my will's in order and if you don't leave me alone, I'll put Star and Craig (Eve's son) in charge of everything." Both boys were 18 at the time. Earlier he'd said he wanted the "60 peso funeral," the cheapest in Mexico!

The last weekend there were fewer people, and we all stayed overnight in our Victoria Street home. The whisperings in the kitchen subsided. It was quiet and everything felt right. John was tending to dying and each of us to finishing in our own way our 'business' with him.

On the day before he died, John asked Dr. Greg if there was any way for him to live. Greg gave the medical answer, "No, we can only make you as comfortable as possible without making you unconscious." John said, "I'm too uncomfortable to go on living anyway."

As Greg left the room, John said to me, "Deborah, you've got to stop your compulsive lying." He had a knack for getting someone's attention by using something they were attached to . . . like my image of myself as an honest person. At first I thought he was referring to my saying "nobody dies" because the doctor had just told him he was going to die. But that wasn't it. I was stunned. I felt I'd been kicked in the gut with a huge boot. I asked him to repeat what he'd said and he did. Choked and teary I said, "Don't you dare die without explaining what you mean. It's not fair to leave a ghost like that." He continued, "Stop saying you're *going* to quit smoking or *going* to do anything in the *future*." What I understood from his slurred words was that he was trying to help me stop setting boobytraps for myself. Often enough he'd seen me project something I might do in the future, then feel I'd failed when I didn't do it. One of his last gifts was again trying to help me live in the *present*.

That night none of us expected John to live till the next day. We held our last healing circle. This time the healing was for John, not for his body. He seemed to finally accept that we loved *him*, not just the part of him that helped us out or made our lives happier. We loved him whether or not he finished his book.

After the healing circle he said, "Eve, I love you . . . such good friends!" And someone said, "You've been a wonderful friend to us." John did not speak again.

We scheduled ourselves by twos every two hours to help him sit up and cough. His breathing by now came and went with a rattle—the sound was unnerving. He could no longer swallow and we kept moistening his parched lips. It was terrible to watch helplessly as he suffered. The shifts shortened to one hour, then to half an hour. When not on shift, we cuddled together like children and slept on mattresses that covered the living room floor. I remember looking down on my sleeping partners and feeling how much I loved them.

John labored all night, coughing and struggling for air. He seemed to want to let go but his body had a life of its own and kept hanging on.

In the morning I went to my construction job, plastering. Rough to get the walls smooth when my heart and mind were with John and the family. Each time I called home, John was still alive. After work I went by the most expensive food store in town and bought two baskets of fresh raspberries and a Toblerone chocolate bar. Perhaps this outer nourishment might ease the inner loss! I ate one whole basket on the way home and saved the other for Eve.

When I got home, John was weaker and Eve was away. She'd gone out in her car to scream and yell and weep. This, along with dancing, usually helped her remain calm. This time she came back angry. "John has pulled us into a terrible sadness trip. He said death is the greatest adventure of them all—he might as well relax and enjoy it!" Gently she repeated this to John and he relaxed and breathed easier. Maybe he'd been waiting to hear from *her* that it was OK to let go.

She left the room and we sat there and ate the Toblerone. A few minutes later Rusty motioned for me to get her. She came and held John's hand. At 3 o'clock in the afternoon, on November 22 at the age of 59, John stopped breathing. Six of us were there; we chanted *Om* as he left his body. (Om is understood by many as the Primal Sound or the sound that connects us to the spirit. It's used particularly by Hindus and Buddhists.)

Someone suggested we massage the points on his hands and feet corresponding to the solar plexus to help free his soul for its journey. Tears of sadness, relief and joy rolled down our faces. We held each other and prayed, each in his or her own way, for his soul to move quickly on. Candles and incense were lighted. Then we dressed him in his favorite blue flannel shirt and a pair of Eve's drawstring pants. His own were now too big. Eve put an *Ojo de Dios* (God's eye) at his head and a child's pinwheel in his hand. Rusty shaved him. John's face seemed to fill out—all signs of pain and struggle gone. His real nobility of heart again came through the old familiar face.

That night we cried and laughed and told stories. I'd be talking with someone with tears running down my face and the next minute we'd both be laughing as we greeted others. Someone on her way to the house when John died said she saw him whooping up and down the foothills on a roller coaster laughing his head off. Friends phoned and were phoned. Eve called Wavy Gravy, a clown, and told him about John's death. His reply was, "Well, it was Patrick Henry's second choice!"

Two friends went off with a bottle of Scotch to build the pine coffin . . . one thumb hammered! The burial laws of New Mexico are very humane. You may bury someone on private property within 24 hours of death if the site is at least fifty feet from water. You need to file a burial certificate and get a body transfer permit, a one-stop operation. Later you note the burial site on the land deed so a highway or something isn't built over the grave. Ken and Barbara offered a weedy little field by their house as a burial site. We decided to plant an orchard there.

The next morning, waiting for the coffin to arrive, many of us felt unfocused, a little like the day after Christmas. We wanted to bury him quickly. We'd had plenty of time to "clear" with John and it was time to move on. I went to buy a cherry tree and a Jonathan apple for the new orchard and flowers for the grave. We arranged for a truck; a hearse didn't feel right. Our impression that John was a giant of a man manifested in a ridiculously large nine-foot coffin. We placed John's body in it on a faded red *serape*. It was a relief now to be outside. The body had begun to smell which wasn't as noticeable outside. (I learned later that the smell was probably from body fluids released after death.)

We followed as the coffin was driven over to Ken and Barb's. We set it up on sawhorses in the field under a clear, early winter sky. People came and looked and cried. Some put things in the box that they wanted to send with John's body: copies of his two books, a piece of jade, a bit of lapis lazuli, a Tibetan mandala, dancing shoes. Carl Franz, author of *The People's Guide to Mexico,* put a pen in John's shirt pocket. "You can't put an author away without a pen."

We dug a great hole in the earth, deeper than it needed to be. Nearly everyone wanted a turn digging. I watched a friend with tears running down his face work with pick and shovel until he was exhausted. "This is the last thing I can do for him." It was great therapy to be out in the fresh air using our bodies. I wondered later why people let professionals take this useful bit of therapy away from them.

We made a large circle, some 60 people, joining hands around the coffin. Whoever wanted to could speak. Eve had asked a friend to read a passage from *The Velvet Monkey Wrench:*

> Imitating someone else's style just because they are stronger, richer, fatter, or hipper is a stone drag. Picking our very own lifestyles is not a process of copying.

Not many of us trusted that if we opened our mouths words would come. Instead we sang *When the Saints Come Marching In,* and two women sat on a knoll playing a french horn and a fiddle. Eve tossed a yellow rose on top of the box for an absent friend as it was lowered into the earth. We shoveled in the earth and planted and watered a Jonathan apple tree.

A friend was free. A new orchard begun. A great day to celebrate . . . feasting, talking, dancing, crying, holding and being held. Ken asked, "Why aren't we this close all the time?"

John's last gift was giving us an opportunity to learn that "Dying is OK."

* * * * *

In many ways, John's experience and ours with him was unusual, but the feelings and situations we encountered are common.

In case you're beginning to feel hopeless and think you can't handle someone's dying without a squadron of 20 friends, buckets of money, an extra house and endless supporters, take a break . . . then read on.

Mary

My next experience with dying came while we were still discussing writing a book about the last one. What we'd learned with John seemed useful to share.

Mary Conley's dying was very different from John's. Cancer was about the only thing they had in common. Mary had few close friends and almost no money. Her wealth was the faith that death is a doorway to more life. The richness of our shared faith, my experience with John, and fewer people to orchestrate made her dying much easier for me.

There were four of us: Mary, her 21-year-old son Craig, myself, and later Craig's friend Jean. At first we felt alone, a tiny island tending to dying in a world going about business as usual. Our combined resources at the time were $200 and a house with one month's rent paid. Neither Craig nor Jean had been in close contact with someone dying, although Mary's husband (Craig's father) had died ten years earlier of cancer. A daughter in Mexico had already done what she could and was not with us. That seemed OK. Each person has to decide what's right for them when someone's dying; not everyone has to be or can be present.

Mary and I met in San Miguel about the same time I met John and Eve and became close and beloved spiritual sisters. After her husband died, she traveled with her children and continued to study astrology and the principles of spiritual life. When we met she was a doting young grandmother often caring for her baby granddaughter by herself while writing a book on the Tarot. The Tarot is an ancient system that uses universal archetypal symbols to bring to the conscious mind what the unconscious mind knows.

When I was especially happy or depressed, I'd head down the cobblestone alleys to Mary's tiny adobe house at the bottom of the hill. No matter what state I arrived in, I left feeling better and seeing my life more clearly. Many others can say the same. Mary shared herself and her wisdom with anyone who arrived on her doorstep and wanted to receive them. Her influence is partially responsible for changing and expanding my vision of who I am.

For two years almost no one knew Mary had cancer. The last year of that time, she was housemother in a home for pregnant teenagers. Mary was the one who held a rejected girl's hand as she went through labor. Mary's love and guidance helped at least 30 young girls live through a fearful experience. And at the same time she was working on healing her own dis-ease.

Mary knew cancer was her teacher and looked for the lessons it offered. She understood life as a spiral of births into flesh and deaths into spirit, moving closer each time to one's God-Self. The teaching now pointed to something she needed to understand for this journey home. Mary believed it was about the fear and unworthiness she felt as a parentless child. Since her childhood she'd struggled between two parts of her personality she called Pitiful Pearl and Mary C. Pitiful Pearl was always afraid and felt she didn't deserve anything good in life. Mary C., on the other hand, was wise and courageous and manifested strongly when she was house-mother. Mary thought that as Mary C. got stronger, Pitiful Pearl felt threatened and expressed herself by creating illness. It seemed to me that not expressing her sadness nor loving herself as generously as she loved others were important factors in her illness. Until the last five months, she seemed to have eliminated the cancer.

Mary's dying began for me with a phone call I received at my parents' home in Texas. Craig said he and Mary were alone in her tiny second-story apartment in Albuquerque and both feeling crazy with the confinement and summer heat. They'd just returned from trips to a laetrile clinic in Mexico and to a psychic healer in Costa Rica and Mary was in terrible shape. I told him, "OK, I'm coming. We'll go to my house in Santa Fe." After I said it, my 'Fearful One' did a terrific dance. How could I care for her and work on my M.A. thesis and make enough money to survive? What if she was in terrible pain and I couldn't help? Where could I move if I had to leave my house because the echoes of her pain were haunting me?

In Albuquerque, I found a tiny, shriveled being who couldn't move or eat alone. When I'd last seen Mary five months earlier she was an attractive, peppery red-haired woman of 50 who looked 40. Now she appeared a gray, skeletal 80. My initial joy at seeing her changed to shock and pain. My chest felt like it was pushed against my spine. We decided I'd go to Santa Fe and clean house, then return for her.

During the hour's drive home, I yelled from as deep in my gut as I could. Yelling relieved the pressure; I was free to race around preparing the four small rooms. I chose the living room for Mary because afternoon sun illuminates it and the mountains, and I needed the nourishing morning light of my bedroom. I moved furniture, hung a wind chime and bird-feeder outside her windows, bought a bedpan and straws that bent, washed and ironed pastel silk nightgowns, rented a wheelchair and potty chair and chose music she might like.

We decided to bring Mary to Santa Fe in a pickup truck because we couldn't afford an ambulance. Craig called the Fire Department Rescue Squad to carry her down the steep stairs of her apartment building. They helped Mary onto the foam mattress in the pickup and we wedged her in with quilts and pillows. Because Craig's truck was threatening to break down, I followed him slowly up the valley between the Jemez and Sangre de Cristo mountains. The trip must have been painful but Mary said with her usual grace, "Oh, it was just fine. Thank God to be home in the mountains."

Somehow we helped her out of the pickup into the wheelchair and into bed. She couldn't raise her arms so nightgowns, silk or not, were out! I felt again the blessed relief I'd felt when John came home. Now Mary was *home* and comfortable and had two people who loved her to do whatever was needed. The house was peaceful—filled with loving new energy and wild gold sunflowers.

Craig was exhausted. He'd dropped out the last quarter of his senior year of college to be with his mother. For six weeks he'd single-handedly fed, bathed and moved her everywhere (even between countries), and had helped her with whatever she needed including enemas. Knowing he'd be able to sleep soundly for the first time in months was very satisfying to me. Although he had to sleep on a sheepskin rug in the prayer room, at least there was someone else to take a turn.

Because we had almost no money, we set about phoning everyone in town we could think of for help. If an agency or office couldn't help, we asked if they knew one that could. We followed every lead to get more laetrile which I felt might help with pain. In a few days we had laetrile and two offers of wheelchairs to replace the rented one. We didn't tell Mary we chose the one from the American Cancer Society. She disliked this group because she felt it was controlled by the medical establishment and drug companies. We found a Visiting Nurse Service which had a grant from HEW to help the terminally ill. They supported our decision to be at home, sent gentle competent nurses to visit twice a week and said we could call at any time.

I knew of another group, called Open Hands, who visit with the elderly, disabled and terminally ill and provide counseling and other supportive services like running errands, bathing, cooking or just being there to talk. They'd spell us if we needed it. We found that Mary was eligible for Social Security and applied (although the money came after she died). We found a County Emergency Medical Fund that would pay any hospital expenses. Shanti, a volunteer counseling group, was willing to send a counselor. The nurse friend who gave John his laetrile shots didn't charge to give Mary hers.

Doctor Greg visited Mary and took care of her the night she went to the hospital and never sent a bill. He even took me to dinner one night when I *had* to get away. Another friend co-signed a bank loan so I could splurge on a color TV. With a TV, Mary could have some variety and diversion when she wanted and I felt freer to do what I wanted. I went to a flower shop, told the florist that my friend was dying and that I wanted to surround her with beauty and didn't have much money. He let me scruffle through the trash cans where the imperfect flowers are tossed and I'd go home with bouquets of yellow roses and delicate white baby's breath.

Our day-to-day supporters were each other, God and a friend of Mary's and mine, Gathanna. The Quimby Center in Alamogordo, New Mexico, and the White Lodge in England, sent spiritual healing and support. One friend came with food, massages, love and recipes. (One of my biggest fears had been what to cook.) Another nourished me by calling to check on how I was doing. Craig's relatives sent love and money and I sold antique clothing off the back porch.

I was surprised how much joy I could find in that little house with my friend dying in the living room. For a few minutes each morning before getting out of bed I meditated on joy and imagined myself as the "joyful servant." I put a sign JOY on the refrigerator door and over my bed to remind me of it throughout the day. As I nurtured my "joyful servant," I experienced more and more that it was a privilege to be there for Mary and to have this opportunity to learn.

I joyed in our talks, watching the birds, daubing on Tea Rose perfume, hearing the wind chime's song, and massaging her. There was joy in our jokes about our spiritual interests or my using her as an excuse to get out of meetings I didn't want to go to—and in our "waltzing." When Mary couldn't walk alone anymore, I held her up under her arms. I'd ask, "Madame, may I have this waltz?" Our silliness let her know she wasn't a burden and helped her release some of the frustration of no longer being able to walk alone.

I took time for myself—for Tai Chi, jogging, paperwork and gardening—and encouraged Craig to do the same. He and Jean went camping for two days and visited with old friends. At 21, Craig and Jean seemed young to be going through this. I would have felt motherly, except they were so sensitive and capable.

When Mary came to my house, she was denying that she would die. The denial continued for about three weeks. Maybe if she took more enzymes, she would throw off the cancer! Maybe a piece of stool was blocking her intestines and not a tumor! Maybe we should put poultices on the huge lump on her leg and open and drain it so it wouldn't poison her body! She needed hope.

Another of Mary's ideas was to take coffee enemas to detoxify her liver, which would eliminate the cancer. (Coffee enemas are sometimes used in alternative cancer treatments to help detoxify the liver, but must be part of a larger healing program.) The plan was to build a bench in my white prayer room and give her the enemas there, close to the bathroom. I hit the wall! I couldn't stand the idea of my sanctuary being messed up, and felt guilty for it. "Deborah, how can you be so persnickety! Those enemas might help Mary live . . . at least they'd support her trying to help herself!" I wasn't compassionate enough with myself to think, *There's some-*

*thing important to me about this prayer room that gives me
the strength to support her through this experience.*

To assuage my guilt about my selfishness, I suggested an
alternative plan, a liver flush commonly used in holistic healing. It's a cocktail of cayenne, garlic, ginger, olive oil and
lemon juice mixed in orange juice to help it down. I mixed
one up, a little heavy on the cayenne, and gave it to Mary.
She took two sips, gagged and said, "It's awful!" and in five
minutes she was shaking, sweating and delirious. I jumped
into the bed and held her, thinking, *Deborah, she's going to
die. You've killed her.* Fortunately for me she didn't die but I
felt guilty anyway. At that time I didn't yet understand the
pattern of guilt enough not to feel it.

About a week before Mary died, lumps sprouted all over
her body. It was obvious she was dying, yet she was still
denying it. Craig often felt disgusted and angry with his
mother's lack of acceptance. He said, "She's denying everything she ever taught me." He wished it were already over
and felt guilty for wishing it. He didn't realize that many
people, living with someone they love who is dying slowly,
have similar feelings. I suggested it was perfectly natural;
guilt was unnecessary. It is possible to feel *"I wish it were
over"* and have compassion at the same time. Sometimes I
was also fed up. I wanted Mary to be somewhere she
wasn't: already accepting her death. That problem was
mine, not hers.

Dealing with our frustrations was more difficult than physically caring for Mary. We'd sit on the back porch watching
the chipmunks play and talk out the things that bothered us.
Sharing this way released a lot of blocked feelings.

After one of these back porch discussions, Craig and I
decided to tell Mary what we thought about her condition.
Our decision grew out of frustration with the attempts to save
her. Doctor Greg wasn't around to talk with her, so I told
Mary, "We feel it would take a miracle to save your body. We
believe in miracles, and also believe it would have to be a big
one . . . soon." This left some room for hope and gave her a
clear picture of what *we* thought was happening.

She decided on a trip to the hospital to find out if some physical or mechanical obstruction, other than a cancerous tumor, prevented her from eating and eliminating. Although we didn't think much of the idea, it wasn't *our* life so we arranged it. This time we had to get an ambulance. The four of us spent one night in the hospital.

When we came home, Mary had to decide whether or not to continue the intravenous feedings that kept her body from dehydrating. Doctor Greg told her what he knew about dehydration. She decided not to continue the IVs, a decision that took great courage. As she said "no," she was also saying, "I know I'm going to die." She chose, in effect, to die of dehydration instead of cancer. It's not a bad way to go. One slips slowly into unconsciousness. The main discomfort is dryness in the mouth.

About five days before she died, Mary accepted what was happening to her body. That ended the depression and we could talk about death and what her work might be on the other side. If possible, she would report to us. We decided to use sunflowers as a sign for communicating after her death. If we were meditating and saw a sunflower, whatever we heard would be from Mary. I've since had a couple of sunflower messages.

Mary told us, "Get ready for Sunday. I'll be leaving." One part of me was irritated. For months I'd planned a retreat in the mountans that weekend with Patricia Sun, a widely-known spiritual teacher and healer. It took a while for me to realize that the most important spiritual teaching for me was going on in my own home. We started to get ready.

I suggested that Craig talk with his mother about anything unclear in their relationship so he wouldn't be left with the "I-wish-I-hads." Mary's daughter called from Mexico. I held the phone. It was a privilege to share that conversation: a mother saying goodbye to a daughter with whom the relationship had not been easy, expressing her love and her understanding of her daughter's absence.

Craig had Mary's land transferred to his name to avoid

lawyers later. Mary had few other material possessions and told Craig what to do with them. She gave me the perfect reminder of common work, a little gold Florentine box with The Prayer of Saint Francis.

I've often wondered how Craig felt as he went to the lumber yard to buy pine boards and quietly set about building a box for his mother on the back porch. He put his heart and hands to making the best box he could, using screws instead of nails so Mary wouldn't hear the hammering. I became the "interior decorator" and for our sake made the inside of the box beautiful with old hand-sewn quilts.

Saturday and Sunday we let the stops out... no more pacing ourselves. At night we slept lightly in my room, with the door open so we could hear her calls or changes in breathing. During the day we were with her constantly. Seven or eight times daily we massaged her back, hands and feet. Touching was among the few things she still enjoyed. It was important for her to know that she was still a person to us and that we weren't too repulsed to touch her lump-covered body. We continued to wash her teeth, bathe her and comb her hair. To alleviate the dryness in her mouth, we used ice chips or held a wet washcloth for her to suck on.

Sunday, while we were practicing sliding a suction tube down the throat of the visiting nurse in case we'd need this procedure, Mary's breathing became very heavy and labored. I thought she was leaving and suggested she move toward the Light and practice letting go. After hardly speaking for two days she managed to get out, "You're rushing me!" We broke up laughing and joked about the rebellion on our hands. Who is to know God's timetable or what unfinished work she had to do on a level beyond our understanding? From that point on she was in and out of consciousness.

She mumbled or mimed to us to turn her in bed about every twenty minutes, which was tiring because she couldn't help at all. Because she couldn't move, eat or drink and her skin was raw, she was in extreme discomfort. We asked if she wanted a shot of Demerol that had been prescribed, and she nodded. Earlier we'd practiced in the kitchen giving shots to a helpless orange. Jean was elected to give the first one because of her greater experience—giving shots to mice in a biology lab! Because Jean and Craig were willing, I didn't have to face my fear of shots . . . this time.

In the beginning we'd been afraid that we might not know what to do for Mary, but as each situation arose, we found we could handle it, which increased our confidence for the next. Taking care of things ourselves seemed preferable to waiting for a nurse.

Demerol was the first pain medication Mary took since way back when she could swallow an occasional Tylenol. In the hospital, doctors and nurses were amazed she wasn't in pain. Perhaps the laetrile helped. Color therapy and Bach Flowers (see Appendices A and B) may also have been a factor in preventing the intense pain one might expect with tumors all over the body and with the vital organs barely functioning.

Monday evening Dr. Greg stopped by and said, "You know, she could go on breathing like this for a couple of days." I crumbled. A few nights earlier he had gently and sensitively given her the talk he gave to John. "We can't save your body, but we'll make you as comfortable as possible." Because we'd stopped pacing ourselves, I was exhausted and didn't know if I could keep going as long as she could. We decided I'd go to dinner with Greg and the next morning Craig and Jean would go for a walk in the hills.

As much as I needed to get away, I didn't enjoy it. I felt divided; half of me wanted to be with Mary. When I got home after midnight, Craig and Jean were just lying down on the floor to rest. "How's it going?" I asked. "We just sat quietly with Mom all evening. She's the same." I went in to see her. She was still breathing but looked already dead. I said offhandedly, "She looks macabre," and went into the bathroom. Craig called and she was gone before I got back to her room. I think at some level she had been waiting for me to get home so Craig and Jean wouldn't be alone.

We stood for a bit, shocked by death, the event we had been anticipating. While it was sinking in, I diverted myself by phoning Greg to tell him Mary was dead and to remember the death certificate. Calmed, I went back to her room. We lit candles, said prayers for her to be on her way, and held each other. Then we dressed her in a favorite peach antique silk and lace nightgown. I tied a scarf from under her chin to the top of her head (as if she had a toothache) so her mouth would set closed. With the focus of our energy suddenly gone, we felt shaky, uncertain. Holding each other and praying helped steady us. We all thought of food at the same time and left the body to go rummage through the refrigerator. How surprising to be hungry! We talked a while, then fell into our sleeping places feeling we could sleep indefinitely.

No. Greg woke us at 6:00 A.M. to certify her death. I could easily have waited till 9:00 to have the obvious officially confirmed. We lifted Mary's body into the coffin which, after all my warnings about John's absurdly big one, seemed to me a little snug. Craig still maintains it was just right. After putting in her Tarot deck, Craig hammered down the top of the box, and he and his childhood friend, Joey, loaded the heavy coffin into my pickup. We were to meet Greg at the Office of Vital Statistics to fill out the death certificate and body transferral form. Mary had wanted to be buried on her land in the mountains three hours north of Santa Fe.

Greg thought our digging crew was understaffed and volunteered to help, but not without breakfast. So while Craig, Joey and Jean set off with borrowed picks and shovels, I had breakfast with Greg. The young doctor told me, "I hope if I help enough folks, there'll be people around to give me a good burial some day."

On the way, I stopped at my usual gas station. The owner asked what I was up to and I answered, "I'm off to the mountains to bury my friend," and motioned toward the back of the truck. The look on his face when he saw the coffin delighted me. Our relationship has been different since that day—he now takes a personal interest in what I carry in the back of my truck.

It was an exquisite late summer day. The high desert country was covered with purple asters, golden chamisa and silver Indian sage. We chose a spot called The Meadow overlooking valleys and more mountains. 'Meadow' in the Southwest generally means open, not green and grassy. This one was covered with gray, weathered wood, sculpted like driftwood. As we dug, Greg took the role of "the one who knows." I let go and was silly . . . and how I needed to be silly.

I shoveled a little, but mostly walked in the wind and felt the joy of being free in the mountains after so many days indoors. The others joked and told stories; dug and rested; ate and drank beer. The hole seemed to keep getting shallower. I kept changing, "Bury me six feet deep in the lone prairie" to "Bury me four feet deep. . . ." Craig wouldn't have it. "The hole has to be deep enough so animals can't dig her up." This seemed unlikely with the top hammered down.

When the sun began to set and we were still digging, I was worried. I was due back in town for a lecture I was co-sponsoring. There was nothing to do now but let go and trust that someone would handle it. We finished digging in the headlight beams of the pickups with the moon already up. I lashed together a cross of four equal arms and placed it in a circle of stones. As I felt the earth in my hands the sense of loss of a sister caught up with me and I cried. Greg squatted beside me and repeated a translation of the Navajo prayer, Beauty Way:

> *May it be beautiful before me.*
> *May it be beautiful behind me.*
> *May it be beautiful below me.*
> *May it be beautiful above me.*
> *May it be beautiful all around me.*
> *In beauty it is finished.*

Dad

Throughout the writing of this book, I knew my father was dying. My friends' deaths and writing this book were part of my preparation to accept his death.

My family is a family like many others—perhaps extraordinary in the amount of love and loyalty among us. Each of us would tell a different story about my father's death. This is mine.

When we found out *we* had cancer, it was not seen as Dad's alone but as the concern of us all.

It was Eastertime and the bluebonnets were blooming when we gathered in San Antonio, Texas, to be with him for his first surgery. We were frightened. When hours and more hours passed and we were still sitting in a waiting room at the VA hospital, we knew the cancer must be more extensive than the surgeons had thought.

Dad came out of surgery into a ward with exceptionally overworked nurses, which made them appear incompetent and unloving. The ward he shared with three other men was like a TV M.A.S.H. unit. The humor in the situation saved us. We were all in the same leaky life boat together!

The chief instigator, a man named Dolph, wore a panama hat with his pajamas, sneaked cigarettes and drank hot coffee right before his temperature was taken. Anything the men needed, except pain medication, we had to do or find. We'd go off "midnight requisitioning," looking through closets for pajamas, sheets, towels, ice, and lemon swabs—the most appetizing items available.

The camaraderie of the four men—a Navy admiral's steward, an Army master sergeant, a warrant officer, and my father, a colonel—helped us adjust to his situation. At times we laughed so hard that Dad had to hold his stitches to keep them from bursting. And the laughter opened our hearts and released some of the pain and fear.

After surgery, Dad's way to treat cancer of the colon was chemotherapy. That was not my way. I'd studied and worked with natural healing and had seen friends heal themselves of cancer without drugs and surgery. Choosing chemotherapy seemed to me like signing a death warrant because it severely damages the body's immune system. I knew Dad had to do it his own way *and* I didn't want him to die! I gave him all the information I had on alternative healing and his response was, "I don't want to be the world's greatest expert on cancer." He had faith in the medical system he grew up with and in a young Dr. Page at the VA hospital. The VA hospital was connected with the University of Texas Medical School and to research programs around the country. One week each month he stayed in the hospital for chemotherapy.

I returned to Santa Fe furious with the medical establishment, which admitted it didn't have the answer but insinuated that its way was the only way. I was furious with the Army for sending human beings, including my father, to be guinea pigs at the nuclear bomb tests in Nevada in the 1950s. I was angry with everything and I hurt. There were lots of summer mornings when I sat on my back porch eating breakfast with tears rolling into my cereal. Slowly, very slowly, what I knew in my head entered my heart. Each of us has to die in our own way. I began to take interest in my work again.

I thought of Dad often that summer as I worked on this book. I remembered him as a father. I remembered him and Mother tucking the twins, Judy and Suzy, and me into bed every night; his singing a song to wake us up for school; his taking me alone to Holland and braiding my pigtails and letting me pick as many tulips as I wanted; teaching us to shoot and hunt; taking us exploring on the weekends, even when we didn't want to go. I remember now his face as I looked up from a wheelchair when he met me and my sheep dog in Mexico the time I came home sick from the diplomatic service in Chile. I remember his voice when I phoned from Mexico to say I'd broken my back, then he and Mother taking turns visiting me twice a day in a hospital in San Antonio—his walking me up and down the halls as I learned to walk again. I remember his wanting to go to New England with Mom to help Suzy when her Joshua was born and instead staying home to take care of my sheep dog. He loved, trusted and was proud of us. The only real gripe I remember was when he said, "Do it right or don't do it at all"—and "right" meant "his way".

Who was this man I loved so much? He was my mother's husband for 43 years. But that's her story. What I know is that the light from their marriage gave other people strength.

Col. Edward Duda was an army officer for thirty years. (My friends would say, "But how can an army officer be so mellow?") What was it like for him after he retired and instead of his telling 20,000 men when to jump, Mother would tell him to put his dishes on the *left* side of the sink? Who was this quiet, charming man who reminded some of Jimmy Stewart, which secretly delighted me? I'd watch him and wonder... He once even said, "I wish you wouldn't watch me so much."

Dad was born a few years after his parents came steerage class on a boat from Poland; they worked hard to make it in a new country. Ethnic groups weren't fashionable at the time and Dad wanted to be an American, not a Pollack kid. He grew up proving a Duda was as good as a Johnson, Jones or Smith. Because the American culture values doing and achieving, he set out to achieve—editor of the yearbook, captain of the track team, the fastest runner ("The Irvington Flash"), senior class president, the Zippity Duda who worked his way through college and graduated with honors. First the Depression, then World War II, made Dad and nearly everyone else think of security. He was called into the army a day after I was born, liked it and stayed. He wanted to be a general. But the army, like every company, has its politics, and he didn't make it. We were proud of him anyway, but I imagine he hurt.

Why the cancer? Why him?

One evening we recorded Dad's life story up to his high school years. One of the first things he remembered was an accident when he was seven. He was relaxed and having fun when a kid hit him in the eye with a baseball bat. From then on, he said, his vision was distorted. Later he related,

> When I was a boy, I believed the most important thing was being in control; if I wasn't, I got hurt. My family got upset when I was hurt. I grew up believing that my being hurt made others suffer ... so when I hurt, I kept it to myself. I kept swallowing the hurt. When I was older, I didn't hurt anymore ... I wouldn't let myself. But things still happened that made me hurt and it just sat inside. I picked up the radiation in Nevada. Without all that hurt, it wouldn't have affected me. The hurt was a weakness the radiation could attach itself to ... the hurt became the cancer.

As a little girl I saw the hurt and decided I had to be Dad's protectress; and now he had cancer and I couldn't protect him. Part of me still wanted to and part of me realized this was his opportunity to learn.

That summer and fall, everything went along fairly smoothly. Mom sent out Christmas cards that said, "We have cancer and we're doing fine." We all wondered if this was the last year Dad would put the angel we'd had for 35 years on top of the tree.

One morning four months later, I woke up in Mexico knowing something was wrong at home and phoned. Mom was crying. Dad was in the hospital again. They'd found a huge tumor in his liver and spots on his lungs and were planning to operate. She'd been sitting up all night alone in the house with my dying sheep dog Benjy, and had just taken him to be put to sleep.

After a series of painful tests, the doctors decided Dad's tumor was inoperable. They decided to insert a tube into the liver so chemotherapy drugs could be fed directly into it, "a minor operation." Mom was holding together pretty well. She'd always said, "I can do anything I have to."

I arrived home in time for surgery. In the waiting room Mom played cards, *I held the Light* for Dad (p. 213) and we picnicked on chicken. The ward room held a strange fascination for me. I watched deserted old and young soldiers sitting in wheel chairs, connected to tubes, many with mechanical voice boxes, watching TV quiz shows while life slowly drained out of them. I remembered Mother Teresa calling loneliness the worst human disease, and I imagined each man filled with love. Focusing on love prevented my worrying about Dad. I ran into the hall when I saw orderlies wheeling him to his room on a stretcher, writhing in pain. That old instinct to protect him welled up and I could do nothing.

After Dad came home we buried Benjy's ashes in the back yard. Dad cried and cried—for himself, for Benjy, for us all. It was the first time I'd seen him cry since he'd found out he had cancer, although Mom said they'd had some good cries together.

Each day we had to flush a solution through the tube in the artery to Dad's liver. If we didn't clamp the tube properly, blood would spurt out all over. After working in the hospital this didn't frighten me. For Mom and Dad it was very unnerving at first. Taking responsibility for irrigating that tube was an important step in increasing their confidence that they could take care of Dad's needs at home.

The talk at home changed from "could he be cured" to "how long he might live." Dad hoped to make it to hunting season and Christmas. Together he and I were learning what Mom seemed born knowing—surrender. Instead of learning it from my friends with their seemingly free lifestyles, I was learning it from this modest middle-class couple who lived in the suburbs. Dad accepted he was dying nearly a year before he died so he was able to live fully his remaining time. Even after he accepted what was happening it took him a while to get used to not being in control.

I returned to New Mexico to continue writing; Suzy and her boys moved to Texas to live with Mom and Dad. Because Dad had chosen chemotherapy, I prepared myself to hear that he'd chosen to die in a hospital. Also, Mother, Suzy and Judy had said they didn't think they could handle his dying at home. Finally I could even accept that dying in a hospital, although contrary to my values, was OK.

In October Mother phoned and remarked as an after-thought, "Oh, your father wants to die at home." At first I was afraid I'd misunderstood—then I was overjoyed. We were going to be home together and care for Dad ourselves! I couldn't wait to get to Texas. The hardest part—accepting that Dad was dying and making the decision where it would take place—was over.

Hunting season began. Dad was weak, in pain and de-termined to go. Each weekend we bundled him up, prepared food he hardly ate, and his friends took him hunting. He sat in the open door of the cabin, a potbellied stove burning behind him; his rifle, now almost too heavy for him to lift, sat on a table in front of him. He didn't shoot a deer . . . and it didn't matter. He was living—enjoying the silence of the country, the companionship of his friends—forgetting for a time he was dying. I'm grateful to those loving men.

When Dad walked out the door, we put him in God's hands and didn't worry about him . . . well, just a little. His weekends away gave Mom and me time to take care of ourselves so we'd have the energy to support him. I didn't have to wait up to make sure he remembered the 11 o'clock pain pills. Mom didn't have to wake up to help give the ones at 3 a.m., or worry about what to serve him for the next meal.

She dreaded figuring out what to feed him. There was little he could eat without gagging or throwing up, a physical problem Mom took personally as a reflection on her ability to nourish. She's a gourmet cook and sharing love with food was no longer possible. It was a painful part of her process of letting go. For those weekends, she wasn't reminded at each meal that he was dying.

When Dad wasn't hunting, he sat in his reclining chair in the family room next to the patio doors. After a morning hug, he read the print off the newspapers as usual, played with the kids, worked on his taxpayer revolt, and directed the finish-ing of the cabin at the river that he and Mom had started to build with their own hands. Mom continued to keep their financial affairs in order. I remember Dad sitting in his chair, smiling and saying, "I feel so healthy I forget I have cancer." He was healthy in his heart.

Neighbors brought over banana pudding, casseroles and roses and prayed for our family. Dad's sister and her husband visited from New Jersey. Auntie Thelma, Mom's sister and our fairy godmother, called long distance twice a week. Friends phoned every day. It was difficult for the ones who visited to see Dad so weak. And it was as hard for them to express their feelings as it was for Dad to express his. Judy would come over after teaching to eat and play cards with Mom. She often felt frustrated at not knowing how to help Dad.

Ben, 4, and Joshua, 9, brought a lot of joy to us all. As kids do, they went about playing as usual. As we shared their play, we'd forget about dying. They knew Gramps was dying and couldn't do all the things he used to do with them and that he was going to die at home. Shining little Ben would come home from school and drop his drawings and lessons on Dad's lap for approval. Ben was learning to read and they'd work together on letters and sounds.

For Joshua, Gramp's dying was harder. He'd recently left his father in Massachusetts and now Gramps was going to leave too. Like his grandfather he had difficulty in expressing his feelings so communicating was difficult. But he agreed with Ben who said, "I like it better when Gramps is home." For his birthday Josh was allowed to pick a dog from the pound. With Dad dying we'd been concerned that a new dog would be just more complication, but when he and Josh enjoyed the dog so much, we wished we'd done it earlier!

At times, we all took it personally when Dad grouched because he was losing control of the few things he still felt he had command over. One night after Mom or Josh was in tears over one of Dad's grouches, I got angry. "Dad, everything that is flexible has to do with life and everything that is rigid has to do with death. If people always have to play or do

things your way, you may end up with no one to play with."
I'd cleaned out my anger and he understood. It was an
accomplishment for me to let him see me angry because he
thought being angry was 'losing control' and he'd never
approved of it.

Unlike Mary and John, Dad had pain that was difficult to
control. The liver tumor expanded until it pressed against the
nerves of the solar plexus. He was depressed because he
constantly hurt physically. I guess he put up with the pain
because he thought pain had to be part of dying. I told him,
"You need your energy to live the time we have. There's no
need to tough out the pain." With his doctor's approval we
upped the Dilaudid from a usually potent 12 mg. every four
hours to even stronger dosages that would have been lethal
for some. Before raising the dosage, we first tried other pain
relief techniques—breathing into the painful area, hot water
bottles on his stomach and/or feet, hot cloths on his forehead. Sometimes we survived a painful period without raising the dosage. He wanted to keep the dosage down because
he didn't like sleeping so much.

For nausea he took Compazine one hour before the Dilaudid, and Ritalin, a stimulant, twice a day to counteract the
sedative action of Dilaudid. For general well-being, I gave
him Bach Flowers and massaged his feet once or twice daily,
and focused on filling him with love.

Although we appreciated having medical support available we needed very little, except for pain medicine and
information about it. We joined the St. Benedict Hospice
Program so if we needed help, it could come to us. The
hospice nurse visited three times, not because we needed
her, but because it was required by the program. It reassured
Dad to question her about his symptoms. It made me laugh
with love to see the family worrying about not hurting the
nurse's and social worker's feelings because we needed so
little outside help. If I hadn't had previous experience with
dying, however, the program would have been invaluable.

Our chief outside supporter was Angie, the cancer research nurse from the VA, who soon became "family." She became personally involved and worked with us as equals. She was the go-between between ourselves and Dr. Page. We phoned her with questions; she got answers, arranged prescriptions and brought us medicines and supplies. This saved us running around when we had little extra energy. Help like hers might be a model for supporting dying without the need for hospitalization.

Angie had me inject a needle into her arm to help me overcome the terror of shots I'd avoided facing with Mary. Because we'd traveled overseas a lot, I felt I'd spent half my childhood hiding under tables from people with needles. And now Dad might need Methadone injections. One day Dad said, "Deborah, I need a shot." I said "OK." Following the instructions in this book, I gave it to him. It was that simple. When I wanted to help him, I forgot my fear.

Another day, at the time of the celebration over the return of the hostages from Iran, Dad was in pain and we'd done everything we knew to do. I hated seeing him in pain and I felt hopeless and beaten. I went off alone and told God, "I've done my best and he's still in pain. He's in your hands. There must be something he has to learn from the pain."

When I stopped being Dad's protectress and accepted his pain (my pain), I felt at peace. Then a new idea came: I'd find some THC, the active ingredient in marijuana. It combats nausea and also reduces the amount of pain medication needed. He chose not to smoke marijuana, but was willing to take socially and legally acceptable pills.

After we gave it to him, Dad became the beaming Buddha. He sat in his chair radiating sweetness, beauty and love. The THC appeared to open his awareness to his own nature and also to undermine his will. And *will* was holding Dad in his body. By Sunday afternoon he was nearly dead. He sat in his chair and looked dead. He could not talk or move.

Suzy, Judy, mother and I gathered around him. With tears running down her face, Mom tried to wake him. She couldn't. *This is it. Dad's going to die now.* We cried and told him we loved him. Mom remembered 'last rites' because Dad was raised a Catholic—and still went to Mass twice a year. Suzy volunteered to find a priest and got on the phone. We were huddled around Dad when we heard her say, "Well, he's *somewhat* Catholic." We all burst out laughing. Tears of laughter mixed with tears of pain.

Neighbors appeared and told Dad they loved him. Someone put a cross beside him and a rosary in his hand. The priest came and went. Dr. Charlie appeared saying he'd just dropped in for a social visit. Actually he'd driven 15 miles because a neighbor had called and told him Dad was dying. Yes, he agreed, Dad was dying. We decided to carry him to his bed.

Six of us had him lifted in the air when Dad opened his eyes and said, "What's going on?"

Dad lived, and actively, another two weeks. He continued to love swinging outside with us in the winter sun, and playing with Joshua's new dog, Pizza. One of our last projects together was to paint Indian glyphs on a deerskin he'd tanned and stretched on a frame. The symbols he chose (three triangles, a man walking with an eagle coming out of his head, the sun and two fish) showed a man dying in peace.

Gradually he needed more attention. He used a cane to walk from the family room to the bathroom, ate almost nothing and often seemed to drift away. He was so skinny that we put a foam pad on his chair and bed at night for comfort and to prevent bedsores. We dropped the schedule for pain medication and played it by ear. We'd discuss the amount he wanted and whether he wanted pills or shots, then arranged a schedule so Mom and I could sleep as much as possible.

Angie asked Dad if he were willing to be interviewed for a newspaper story on dying. Talking used a lot of energy but Dad said, "Fine, if it will help someone." The reporter asked how he'd decided to die at home. He said, "I knew Debby's friends who died and their way sounded more like the way I wanted to go. I'd read her manuscript and heard about the hospice idea. I saw friends, fellow cancer patients, dying in the hospital . . . it seemed such an ignominious death.''

The reporter asked Mom how she felt when Dad said he wanted to die at home. ''If he was happier at home, we'd work it out. . . I couldn't have done this alone.''

What about joy and dying? Dad answered, ''Well, at least you don't have any more problems!'' He and Mom both said, ''We don't know about joy but we do feel peace.'' *After you were diagnosed, how long was it before you could accept you were going to die?* ''Well, I was shocked. I felt angry and afraid and 'why me,' all those things you read about. Right after I heard I had cancer, I ran into a doctor who gave me hope. He told me it wasn't the end; his mother was a healthy 86 and had had cancer for years. I held onto 'It's not the end.'

''I'd like to tell people not to be afraid of dying. Dying gave me a chance to get rid of sadness and feel peace. You can combine dying with your ordinary life. And doctors and nurses can help us get over the gap before we realize we can live while we're dying.''

A few days after the interview Dad said he didn't feel like walking to his chair. He stayed in bed except to go to the bathroom. Friends brought over foam wedges to prop up his legs to take pressure off his swollen ankles. Josh brought in his little TV.

That night we knew time was running out . . . and that it didn't exist. Mother and Dad rested together on their bed, leaning against each other. The beauty and peace in their faces spoke of the long journey shared together . . . and of the shared journey of all people. And love had made it worthwhile.

The next morning was sunny and springlike for February. I was happy padding around barefoot in jeans shaving and bathing Dad. We were alone. Mom had secretly gone to check out funeral homes; Suzy was working on the first issue of the newspaper she was starting; the kids were at school. Dad and I had a beautiful talk.

He already knew I didn't believe death was the end; that

we just leave a body that is no longer useful to us. We'd talked before about reincarnation and my remembering our being together in other times. This time we talked of preparations. I told him about spiritual teachings that suggest that when you feel yourself lifting out of your body, keep repeating 'God' and follow the brightest light. Dad *heard* me and repeated, "OK, remember to say 'God' and follow the light."

Our talk ended when Dr. Page arrived with Angie for a social visit. Dad was pleased Dr. Page cared enough to come and that he hadn't been just another number in the VA mill. Mom asked Dr. Page the old question, "How long?" He said, "two days, two weeks!" I knew that was inaccurate.

We spent that evening around his bed. Dad played with Ben—rolling up a magazine telescope to watch him play hide-and-seek with himself. Josh said goodbye on his way out to Cub Scouts. Dad and I watched the world news to see if Poland was being invaded as Mom worked on her Saturday Review "double crostic." Dad gave us instructions on the light fixtures at the cabin and on giving away his hunting guns. Suzy came in; he told her he loved her and repeated how much he loved us all. He considered phoning to ask Judy to come but decided it would worry her. "I'll *probably* be here in the morning."

Angie came in about 9:00 p.m. out of a howling wind and rainstorm that the morning sun had never announced. After she took his vital signs, she asked if she could stay over and sleep on the couch. While we sat around him visiting, Dad was looking at himself in the mirror across the room. Suddenly he started and asked, "Do you see what I see?" I said I saw light all around him. He said he saw white light and rainbows, and when he saw the light, he knew he would die soon.

I asked again if he wanted me to call Judy and he said "yes." Judy came over and they joked together. "I love you, Judy," he told her. She said a teary goodbye. We kissed him goodnight and he didn't speak again.

Mom and I were with Dad when he stopped breathing, a

few hours past midnight on Wednesday, February 11. He was 68. Momma cried as she tucked the covers around him and said, "I love you, Daddy." I 'held the Light' as best I could. I cried as I'm crying now as I write.

I walked out into the dark and wind and down the front yard path beside the stretcher with Dad's body. *"What is it to die but to stand naked in the wind and melt into the sun" (The Prophet).* The ambulance awaited. "I love you Pappa . . . stay with the brightest Light."

I went back to the house and Mom and I crawled into her and Dad's bed. I heard Dad telling me, "If you hurt, let it out. Don't hold on until the pain cripples your will to live." I took time just now to cry again as I did that night. This time I lay on the floor beating it with my arms, kicking, crying and howling to release the pain from my body. I heard a trapped animal freeing itself . . . myself.

That night Mom held me as I cried. Now I am alone with the beating of my heart—a heart opened wider after releasing the pain.

In the morning I *needed* to clean. I washed clothes with a fervor while Judy, Suzy and Mom went to the funeral home. Dad wanted a military funeral with a G.I.'s wooden box. This funeral home had no simple wooden coffins so they chose a grey metal one. They arrived home saying, "It's a good thing you weren't there." (Precisely why I hadn't gone.) We joked about my idea of using an ice pick to punch holes in the box so earth could return to earth more quickly.

The next day was a blur. I planned the eulogy I would give at the funeral service. I'd asked Dad's permission and he said, "OK, but keep it short." Suzy and I had the biggest fight we'd ever had. It grew out of unexpressed pain; neither of us felt appreciated by the other. All my clothes were at the cabin so I huffed off to buy something to wear. After Suzy's lectures on not always doing things my way, I thought maybe I should wear something conservative, not my usual style. Here I was making a production over what to wear. Unbelievable!

At one point I was standing in total despair in a shop door, when a saleslady asked if she could help. "I need a dress for my father's funeral." She said, "Oh yes, black." And I said, "Oh no, white, purple or peach!" I found a floaty peach dress that looked like "me," but chose a purple one so Mom and Dad's friends wouldn't be shocked. At home I told the story to Mom who suggested, "Why don't you go back and get the peach one if it makes you happy?" I was repeating the same old lesson: In the *long run,* doing what you *want, instead of what you think you should,* as long as you take responsibility for it, makes everyone happier.

The next morning I'm not sure if I steeled or centered myself to prepare for limousines, flower wreaths, all the funeral trappings. Last thing out the door Mom joked, "Have you got an icepick?"

Joshua, who'd practiced reading the Twenty-Third Psalm the night before, backed out at the last minute. The part of me that was afraid to speak in public wanted out too. The rest of me wanted everyone to know Dad was alive and free.

With Dad's flag-draped coffin in front of me, I spoke shakily,

> My father is not dead. In this box in front of me lies only a shell. He's free and whole . . . Will you make today a day of joy and celebration as well as sadness? . . . Dad said, "I'm not happy about dying and I'm not afraid . . ." He believes we'll be together again . . . His cancer was a kind teacher. It gave him time to learn and to get his life in order . . . time to prepare for death. It taught him to give up control and surrender . . .
>
> Dad's death is a victory. He chose how he'd die. He chose to accept death, to accept life. Since he lives in our hearts, it's impossible to lose him.

Mom, Ben and I went back a few weeks later to put daisies on his grave: We all knew he wasn't there. I held Mom's hand and read:

> *Do not stand at my grave and weep;*
> *I am not there. I do not sleep.*
> *I am a thousand winds that blow.*

I am the diamond glints on snow.
I am the sunlight on ripened grain.
I am the gentle autumn's rain.
When you awaken in the morning's hush,
I am the swift uplifting rush
Of quiet birds in circled flight.
I am the soft stars that shine at night.
Do not stand at my grave and cry:
I am not there. I did not die.
                    —Anonymous

Ben and I sang "Zippity Duda."

Called or not called, God is always here.

—Carl Jung

Chapter 2

Making the Decision to Die at Home

"Everything can be taken from a man but one thing: the last of the human freedoms—to choose one's attitude in any given set of circumstances, to choose one's own way."

—Victor Frankl, author of
Man's Search for Meaning, and
survivor of Auschwitz and Dachau

When we can no longer control the circumstances of our lives, we can still choose our attitude toward the circumstances. We can do this with dying. We can choose to see dying as a tragedy, teacher, adventure, or simply as an experience to be lived. Our *attitude* will determine the nature of our experience. An optimist and a pessimist see the same world, only through different lenses (attitudes). And as Norman Cousins said, "Pessimism is a waste of time. No one really knows enough to be a pessimist."

When we choose to surrender to life, we choose to be free; and in choosing freedom, we remain in control. This paradox is at the heart of our existence.

To surrender and to be free we have to accept life as it **is** instead of holding on to how we **think it should be.** We can't change something we don't first accept. Surrender and acceptance are not to be confused with resignation and succumbing. Resignation and succumbing are *passive*—something just overpowered or overcame us and we had no choice but to give up.Resignation is self-pity and believing the illusion that we're powerless. On the other hand, acceptance and surrender are positive acts. "I *choose* to let go, to give up control and accept life as it is. And there will be things I can change and things I can't."

If we deny dying and death, we're prisoner to them. When we accept them, we're free *and* regain the power lost in resisting them. We let go of our resistance by *letting go*. It's easy to do and can be hard to get ready to do. The choice to let go must be made in the *heart*. A choice made only in the head, unsupported by the body, feelings and soul, is unlikely to be carried out. If we can remember that choice of attitude, the ultimate freedom, is always available, we make a spacious place in which to experience dying. We can be free whether we are dying ourselves or sharing in the dying of someone we love. We can be free whether we die at home or in a hospital. Choosing our attitude is easier at home than in an atmosphere that unconsciously says dying should be isolated from life and is, therefore, not OK.

As our Western culture emphasized control over nature, death became the uncontrollable enemy. We gave doctors the responsibility for combatting this enemy. Death became increasingly a medical "problem" instead of a natural event. We gave away the responsibility for death (and life) to experts outside of ourselves—big institutions and big business. Until very recently life-sustaining technology said a good death is a hospital death and an unobstructed natural death is euthanasia. And people seem to feel that because they invented the machines, they have to use them. So life ends up not to be for living but to justify machinery. We have become medical consumers.

Ivan Illich, in his book *Medical Nemesis* (a scholarly and intriguing history of attitudes and practices about death), calls death "the ultimate form of consumer resistance." Illich goes on to say, "Today the man best protected against setting the stage for his own dying, is the sick person in critical condition. Society, acting through the medical system, decides when and after what indignities and mutilations he shall die." In the face of death we feel powerless. This doesn't have to be. We're not dying to make doctors and hospitals happy or rich! We begin now to take back what is rightfully ours—our life and our death. Once we gave the medical industry responsibility for our deaths, it became an act of personal courage to die at home. Now more and more courageous people are saying, "I don't want to go away to die. I want to die at home."

State and federal governments are financially supporting more home health care. Insurance companies are adding more home health care benefits to their services. Hospices that care for the terminally ill are developing all over the country. We are returning to dying at home — the old, natural way which most of the world never questioned.

We have a right to die with dignity. Dignity in the dictionary means "worthiness." To me it means *doing things in our own way*. Dying at home we maintain the ability to choose our own way, whether it be a little decision like what time we eat, or a big one like whether or not to use life-sustaining techniques.

We have a right to die with *respect—to see and to be seen*. At home a person remains an individual, rather than "the patient in Room 204B."

Dying at home, we can influence the quality and the quantity of our lives.

Why Die at Home?
The Advantages

(You may want to share this list with the dying person.)

1. It's natural.
2. The dying person can influence the quality and quantity of his or her own life.
3. Respect and dignity are maintained.
4. The dying person feels wanted.
5. You feel useful and needed.
6. The continued presence of love supports you both.
7. You both can live more normally and fully.
8. You can both have more freedom and control. The dying person can tell you what he or she wants. (No one is awakened at 5:45 a.m. for temperature taking or the 20th blood sample.)
9. The dying person can teach you something about living.
10. Home is more supportive of the shift from *curing* to *making comfortable*.
11. In a familiar (and secure) outer environment, both of you have more time for the inner preparations for death.
12. There is time and a place to express feelings of grief, anger and love, so accepting this death and death in general will be easier.
13. When physical death occurs, there's time to experience what's happened without the body being whisked away to make room for the next patient.
14. There's no travel wear and tear between home and hospital. (No worry about loved ones driving at night in bad weather.)
15. You both can see or create your own version of beauty, not institutional green walls.
16. Food at home can be fresher and more nutritious.
17. Living at home costs less.
18. Be it a slum or a palace, it's home!

I met a lovely 92-year-old Spanish lady in the hospital who sat in a wheelchair hooked to tubes, babbling, mostly incoherently, about her bedspread at home, the curtains and the good milk. It seemed to me she was still expressing what she wanted most—to be home. Home is a magic word.

When Is It Not Appropriate to Die at Home?

1. When the dying person doesn't want to.
2. When the family would be too upset to be able to care for him or her.
3. When the hospital can provide services that improve the *quality* of a person's life.
4. When the dying person wants to be hooked into intravenous feedings (IVs), etc., and you can't afford a regular nurse.
5. When there is no one at home to care for the person and you can't afford to pay someone. This may not be a real obstacle. There are hospices and visiting nurse groups with grants to help the terminally ill (see pages 75 and 76).
6. It *may* not be appropriate if there are small children in the family who also need care; not because it wouldn't be good for them to be present, but because you might not be able to manage it all. (If you can't get sufficient extra help at home, a residential hospice program may be a solution—see page 75).
7. If the person plans to donate organs for transplant the death would need to take place in a hospital because the organs are transplanted soon after death.

Making the Decision

Sometimes it's very clear-cut. The person who is dying says, "I want to die at home" or just, "I want to go home." If this happens, you, the family, can discuss among yourselves whether or not this choice will work for everyone concerned. Your preferences, as well as the sick person's, need to be considered. The decision to come home must be a joint one. Only a family that **wants** someone to come home can give the care needed.

More often the situation is not so clear. The sick person still may hope to get better and may well do so. Or, someone may not know or *want* to know how sick she or he is, and feel anxious, afraid and confused. And family and friends may feel the same. It's hard to feel clear about dying when we're getting a morass of conflicting reports from different parts of ourselves; body, mind, feelings and soul each report their own story or reality.

In the face of death, the rational mind is afraid because it can't understand or control what's happening. It *thinks* death is the end and fights it. The body's job is to stay alive. It *senses* that death means extinction and fights it. The feelings (emotions) *feel* confused because their work is to react to the other parts. Evidently, it is the soul, or consciousness, that endures. It seems to make an arbitrary decision to leave, which instigates death, and then can't understand why body, mind and feelings resist and make such a fuss.

No wonder we feel confused by dying and death and often wonder what the heck is going on.

Only the heart is not confused. It *knows* the larger plan. It intuitively knows the whole. It *loves* each part and understands the sacredness of each. It *sees* the truth: life without the lens of fear. When we accept all the parts of ourself— surrender—the heart opens, the conflicting reports end, and we can live fully with dying. Mind, body, feeling and soul are aligned so we can make decisions based on all of our needs.

If this feels like a tall order for you now, keep in mind it can take lifetimes to accept ourselves fully. We can practice by surrendering for brief moments at a time.

Give loving support and information to help everyone involved make the best decision possible at this time. Include in the information what you *want* to do, finances, your own state of health, child care and the availability of nursing help. To avoid exhaustion, I recommend there be at least two people at home to take turns supporting the dying person. In the following section on *Financial Considerations* and in Chapter 3, you'll find more information to help with the decision.

Probably you will want to discuss the choices with a doctor. Remember, a doctor in this circumstance is a provider of information, not a decision-maker. She or he is used to recommending the hospital for very sick people. If a hospital is recommended, ask how it can serve the dying person besides prolonging life. (In Chapter 4, there's information on finding a doctor if you don't already have one.)

A decision need not necessarily be permanent. If a person is home and you still have doubts or it's not working out, a hospital, hospice or nursing home is always available. Returning someone can be emotionally difficult for all concerned, and it's sometimes necessary. Respect your feelings. **You are just as valuable as the dying person.**

Examine your motives carefully before bringing someone home. If guilt is the motive ("If I were a good person, I'd bring her home" or "I *should* bring him home"), you probably won't have the energy to keep going until the person dies. Love sustains us; guilt drains us.

Resentment begins with feeling or thinking that someone *should* do or be something they aren't. "He *should* be cooperative" or "She *should* feel grateful." Keep in mind that people bring the same characteristics to dying as they do to living. A person with a difficult or demanding personality generally dies true to character. Although the process of dying may transform a personality, it would be foolish to expect it. **Do you want to care for the person just as she or he is now?** If you do, you will generally be able to meet the challenges. There will be challenges, and each is an opportunity for growth.

Pain management is one of the great fears of the dying and their families. **In most cases pain can be alleviated just as well at home as in the hospital.** I suspect that dying people living at home have less pain than those in a hospital. Love is a very effective pain neutralizer. If the dying person cannot take pills or liquids, a nurse can give injections or you can learn to give them yourself. With a nurse's help even IVs can come home. **Pain control isn't something to fear; just something to do.**

Another fear of a dying person is, "What will happen to my family?" When he or she sees you at home coping and handling well this terminal illness, the fear will be alleviated.

Dying people fear being a burden. Reassure them they're not and that their dying is part of the whole family's life. For example, when I suggested I come home while Dad was dying, Mom said, "But you've got to get on with *your* life, Deborah." My response was, "What happens in my family *is* part of my life."

You might say to someone who fears being a burden, "Allowing ourselves to receive love and caring is just as important as giving them. Are you going to give the pleasure and privilege of caring for you to your family or to strangers?"

Dying people as well as a lot of the rest of us fear loneliness and being deserted. In Malcolm Muggeridge's *Something Beautiful for God,* Mother Teresa says:

> I have come more and more to realize that it is being un-wanted that is the worst disease that any human being can ever experience... For all kinds of diseases there are medicines and cures. But for being unwanted, except there are willing hands to serve and there's a loving heart to love, I don't think this terrible disease can ever be cured."

Bringing dying people home reassures them they're wanted and won't be deserted. And we may have to reassure them many times. Being at home alleviates loneliness.

Dying people fear losing control over their lives. In the hospital, the staff takes over and largely dictates what the patient can and must do, when you can see them, etc. You and the dying person don't have time to adjust gradually to loss of control. At home, on the other hand, you can take a few steps at a time toward giving up control which makes accepting what's happening—surrender—easier.

The feeling of being totally wrenched by an unnatural catastrophe, common in sudden deaths and many hospital deaths, is less likely to occur at home. You know you're doing all you can do. If the thought comes up afterward, *Maybe I could have done more,* you're likely to let go of it much more quickly than if you'd been isolated from a loved one in a hospital. After caring for someone who dies at home more people report feeling peace as well as loss—a feeling of appropriateness and completion and a greater openness to the new life ahead. Mom said, "I feel good because Dad was so happy to be at home and die the way he wanted to."

Sometimes the dying person is medically termed 'unconscious' and has earlier expressed a desire to be home or has signed a "living will." A living will is a document we can sign any time in our adult lives instructing physicians to withhold or withdraw extraordinary life-sustaining procedures during a terminal illness (see page 201).

Patients whose level of consciousness is uncertain may still let us know what they want. You can ask, for example, "Do you want to go home? Squeeze my hand for 'yes'—blink for 'no.'" Use whatever signal you can invent that uses abilities the person still has available.

Few people realize we have the legal right to leave a hospital without a doctor's approval. A family has the legal right to make a decision for a person who is "incompetent" (not able to make or express his or her own decisions). Under these circumstances, the next of kin can take responsibility for checking the patient out of the hospital. You may be asked to sign a form stating that the patient is leaving the hospital against "medical advice." Attending physicians most frequently just drop a case if they don't agree, but they can resort to legal proceedings if they feel it's not in the *best interest* of the patient to leave. This is uncommon.

Mrs. Henry W. Levinson, Executive Director of Concern for Dying, an educational council, says:

> Theoretically, the patient has the right to be wherever he or she wants to be. However, in case of incompetence of a patient, the institution can put up all kinds of roadblocks and often does. If the family is willing and able to stand firm on their right to make decisions for next of kin, one good position is, 'You required consent before you could treat this patient. We are now refusing that consent and any further treatment of this patient will be without consent and will be considered assault and battery.' If the hospital is not allowed to treat a

patient, generally the hospital utilization review committee will say that the patient can no longer stay in the hospital. On occasion, a doctor or hospital lawyer will feel strongly about the patient's need for treatment or disagree so strongly with the family's decision that they will ask for a court order for the appointment of a guardian for the purpose of treating the patient without the consent of next of kin. These cases are few and far between, however, and the majority of them involve minors.

What is the *best interest* of a person who cannot express his or her own wishes? This is a difficult one. What is the quality of life of someone in a coma, sustained by tubes, with little chance of functioning alone again? What is in the best interest of a patient who expresses a desire to go home and the doctor disagrees?

Here, some profound thinking is necessary about the *quality* of life versus the *quantity*. In a hospital a person may be kept alive longer, but in what condition? What is the difference between a coma in which consciousness lifts out of the body to allow the body to restore itself and a coma in which consciousness leaves to prepare the body for death? When does physical survival cease to be a desirable goal? Each case is different. I believe answers come from an inner or higher source which we can reach through prayer or meditation.

Keeping in mind the considerations I've mentioned that are relevant for you, why not gather as a family to discuss the idea of bringing or keeping someone at home? After this meeting, each individual separately can pray, meditate, think and feel about the choices. At least sleep on it overnight before coming together again to share your preferences. If your decision is "home," affirm it together as a group, recognizing that you may still have doubts and that together you'll do your best. Not everyone has to do everything; one person may want to physically care for the person, another may prefer caring for the children. Remember you're a team.

This could be a good time to make an agreement that may save needless suffering later. It can happen that a medicine or something else we give someone speeds up their process of leaving the body. We cannot know the effects on each individual of all foods, medicines and treatments. Affirm together that if a person dies as a result of something you administer with the *best intention,* there is no need to feel guilty or place blame. God or the mysterious and subtle workings of the universe simply used you to help that person out of their body at that time. *You are aligned with your purpose:* allowing someone to die at home with love around them. If this responsibility is too heavy for you to handle, a nurse may be hired.

In this gathering of family and friends, you may want to express your love and support for each other. Sharing loving energy will strengthen each of you. Whoever *needs* to share in this dying is who needs to be present for it.

Once you've made the decision for *home,* keep in mind that your focus shifts from *curing* to making *comfortable.* Now, do everything possible for comfort rather than to prolong life, as long as the dying person is in agreement. A dying person may want to prolong life for some reason or other. People do change their decisions.

Financial Considerations

Finances probably will be a factor in your decision to experience this dying process at home or in a hospital. **It is generally less expensive to die at home.** John and Mary had few additional expenses, and my father had none.

To keep or bring a dying person home, there must be someone to care for him or her. If you're working, can you arrange leave from work? Can you afford to? Can you work part-time? Can you pay a nurse or doctor if they're needed? Compare these home care costs with hospital costs that are not covered by insurance. Is the person eligible for federal or state disability payments, social services or veterans benefits?

Let's start with **insurance**. Check your policy if you have one. What coverage is provided for home nursing services or doctors' visits? Insurance often covers 80% of the cost after a $100 deductible or 100% after $1,000. What are the limitations on home care services? Just about all policies specify a maximum number of visits covered. If the policy is written in Greek, call an insurance agent, explain what you're considering and ask him or her to explain the benefits to you.

There is a general movement among U.S. insurance companies toward more home health care coverage. New Mexico recently passed a law requiring insurance companies operating there to offer benefits covering home care. The person responsible for insurance claims in the largest visiting nurse service in New Mexico said that Prudential, Equitable, Travelers and Aetna provide good home coverage and that Blue Cross/Blue Shield is more difficult. They require not only that a doctor order services but also that these services be pre-authorized by Blue Cross/Blue Shield.

Medicare and Medicaid cover home care if there is a medically established need for "skilled" services. The aid must be given by a *certified* home health care agency under a doctor's direction. Both programs require an "assessment visit" by a registered nurse. Medicare also covers homecare support provided by a certified hospice (see p. 75).

Depending on your needs, check the availability and costs of hospice and/or nursing services, physical therapists, home health care aides or social workers in your area. For example, in Santa Fe in 1984 our non-profit Visiting Nurse Service charged $55 for a visit by a registered nurse. Visits by a hospice nurse may cost nothing or be reasonably priced. Look under "Nurses" in the yellow pages and talk with a hospice or visiting nurse service in your community. Call your county government to check if they have a Public Health Nurse who makes home visits without charge.

In 1984, the largest visiting nurse service in New Mexico charged $16.50 per hour for a visit by a Registered Nurse, who starts IVs and gives intravenous injections. You may not need one. A Licensed Practical Nurse with general nursing skills cost $12.50 an hour. Nursing assistants providing personal care such as baths and Homemaker Aides to do housekeeping chores and run errands were $8.00 an hour.

Costs vary by area, of course, and by the degree of havoc wrought by inflation. Talk with the nursing service about your **needs** and **resources.** Unless you're working and need a full-time nurse, a nurse can train the family in ordinary nursing skills so you need call only in the event of unusual challenges. In many cases only a few short visits are necessary. Mary had about six visits; Dad had three.

The price of a doctor's visit varies too. Call and ask. Again, let a doctor know your needs and resources. You may not need a visit by a doctor or nurse. We didn't with Dad although some visited for reasons other than need for their professional help.

Hospital costs are insane. John's hospital stays, including two operations but not the doctors' bills, cost $15,000. A 1982 study by the Equitable Life Assurance Society gives the following *daily* charges for a hospital *room:*

	Private	Semi-Private	Intensive
San Francisco	$315	$320	$806
Atlanta	167	158	407
Albuquerque	183	167	470
New York City	349	276	463
Columbus, Ohio	178	139	480
San Antonio	147	121	262

These charges are before they stick the first needle into you! Other hospital costs, such as testing and doctors' visits, are just as variable and expensive.

Nursing homes are less expensive than hospitals but not cheap. For example, in Santa Fe a nursing home runs from $30 to $86 a day for a double with board, which is lower than most places. The charge includes routine nursing, but not supplies used or even laundry.

To give you some idea of what a home-dying can cost, here are the costs for Mary, John and my father. You'll see they varied a lot. Mary had no insurance and practically no money. Her last month at home cost us $600 (of which $350 was for laetrile). One day in the hospital cost $344 and was paid by the County Indigent Fund. A $55 phone bill was paid by Social Security. A $70 bill to a doctor who looked at Mary for three minutes and said, "Yes, she'll die soon" was returned with a note saying we had no money and I hoped his family wasn't hungry. We didn't have to pay $150 for six nursing visits because the agency had an HEW grant. John's three weeks at home cost about $1500, which included $650 for laetrile. My father was covered by the military. His last month cost us nothing beyond the usual expenses of running a home. All his medications were free from the VA hospital.

For further information on financial help, check the following sections in Chapter 3: City, County and State Services; Social Security; Veterans Administration; Home Aides; and Visiting Nurses.

Serving humanity is recognizing our common divinity.

—Phoebe Hummel

Chapter 3

Sources of Help

In one morning on the telephone you can find out a lot that will help you make your decision or, if you've already made it, get you started finding the help you need. Here are the sources I found. You'll find others. New alternatives and possibilities spring up every day.

If someone says, "No, we can't help," ask if they know who can. Keep a list of the useful numbers by your phone. When Mary was dying, we had a bowl on the kitchen table where we put all those little notes we wrote about possible help. Share with the dying person what you find out unless it's clearly inappropriate.

You may not need much help, but you may feel more comfortable knowing where to get it if you need it in a hurry.

Family and Friends

Family and friends may be your biggest help. Let them know that this person they're close to is sick and probably dying, that you're planning a home death, and ask if they're willing and able to help. You do them a favor by offering the opportunity to give of themselves and to face their own fears about dying.

People basically love to help and to feel needed. You might be giving someone who at that moment is experiencing life as meaningless an opportunity to find meaning. There's no need to think you're imposing by asking; everyone is free to say "no." Present a clear opportunity to which "yes" or "no" are equally valid responses. For example, "John is dying at home and we need help running errands, cooking meals, caring for him, etc. Is this a time in your life when you can help?" Let them know you're aware that there are times when it's not possible, and that's fine. It may happen that some of your inner circle of friends move to the outer circle and people you hardly knew before move to the inner.

You may even find a doctor or nurse among family and friends, or be referred to one.

Another idea is to form a neighborhood co-op to care for the sick and dying, a Caring Network. It would take a fair amount of courage for the first person to reach out but it could totally change our feeling of separateness—living isolated lives in city apartments and suburban homes. Starting a caring co-op might take just one phone call to those neighbors you don't know or one meeting at your house to ask for help. It might be organized around your husband, wife or child, then spread to include everyone in the neighborhood. Mrs. Blossom can come over for an hour and sit with John. Julie could come for an hour after school and tidy up. Mr. Smith can mow the lawn. Mrs. Martinez can't come over but can bake a casserole. The Dudas could have the kids over to play. Mr. and Mrs. Levy can come sit with John and watch TV while you get away to the movies. Imagine what would happen to a neighborhood or an apartment house with everyone cooperating, feeling needed, having a sense of purpose and learning to love each other. What a joyful prospect.

Medical and Home Care Help

HOSPICES

If there is a hospice program in your area, you may have to look no further. Even if it is fully booked or still in the process of organizing, they know the services available in your community.

Hospice is a newly popular movement as well as theory about health care. According to Dr. Sylvia A. Lack, a national hospice organizer, "The main concern of a hospice program is the management of terminal disease in such a way that patients live until they die, that their families live with them as they are dying . . . and go on living afterwards."

A care-giving team and volunteers are personally involved with the terminally ill patients and their families. The team generally assists the family in caring for the patient at home. Some hospices have a facility with a homelike, loving atmosphere. The emphasis is on alleviating pain and making the patient and family comfortable psychologically. Sophisticated pain control techniques allow most patients to enjoy their remaining time pain-free and alert.

The first U.S. hospice was started in 1971 in New Haven, Connecticut and was modeled after St. Christopher's Hospice in England. Now more than twelve hundred groups in the U.S. are developing the idea of hospice care. A federal law providing Medicare coverage for home care and bereavement support in certified hospices on a three-year trial basis began November 1983. Hospice services may also be covered by insurance benefits and, if not, are reasonably priced.

Because of its new popularity, the term *hospice* is sometimes misused. Find out exactly the kind of services and atmosphere being offered.

If you're not sure if there's a hospice in your area, check the phone book, call your hospital or the National Hospice Organization—(703) 243-5900. New ones begin frequently.

VISITING NURSES

To locate a nurse, look in the yellow pages under "Nurses" or "Nursing Services." Call the organizations in your area and compare their costs and qualifications. Don't forget to check if your county has a Public Health Nurse who makes home visits.

A visiting nurse can teach you basic nursing skills that relate to providing comfort, moving a patient, changing sheets, bathing and exercising. They can show you how to give non-intravenous injections and advise on feeding problems, enemas and other patient needs. They can answer the patient's questions and recognize when a doctor is needed.

HOME — HEALTH CARE AIDES

Another important kind of assistance comes from Home-Health Care Aides. Their services may include personal care, homemaker, transportation and escort, companionship and counseling. Their training, supervision and cost vary so check around. Aides are not licensed but may have completed a 60 hour training program. To find an aide, call a medical social worker at a hospital to recommend an agency. Look in the yellow or white pages under *Homemaker-Home Health Aide Services, Visiting Nurse Associations, Family Service Agencies* or *Social Service Agencies.* For Further information contact the National Homecaring Council, 235 Park Avenue South, New York, NY 10003.

HOSPITALS

A hospital is always available if you need one. You can use one for particular services, even though the intention is to die at home. If your patient does have to go into a hospital for some treatment that will improve the quality of life, I recommend not leaving him or her there alone. Nurses, no matter how excellent, don't have time to attend to all the emotional and physical needs of their patients. If you do have to leave someone, however, don't feel guilty. They'll manage.

Even if you don't use a hospital, you can call the hospital's Director of Nursing Services for information about other services in your community.

Financial Help

CITY, COUNTY AND STATE SERVICES

Financial help is offered to individuals and families at city, county and state levels. The names of the departments providing funds vary from area to area. Some of the names used are: Health, Health Services, Social Services, Welfare, Human Resources, and Human Services. Look in the white pages of the phone book under the name of your state, county or city. Often there's a central *information number* that can direct you to the right department. If you have trouble locating a service, call the county courthouse.

States administer federal programs such as Medicaid and Aid to Dependent Children.

It can be a headache finding someone in state or local governments who knows more than their little piece of the pie. However, there generally is someone and with perseverance you'll find him or her.

For example, after much calling around I found a woman in our county Social Services office who knew what help was available. She told me about a county emergency relief fund which pays hospital and nursing home bills, and about food stamps, daycare service for children, homemaker service for light housework, a group which does heavy work like cutting wood, and a rent subsidy program. These services are generally *free* if your income is below a certain level, or the fees may be on a sliding scale. In our county there's even an adult protection service which helps people who are confused or incapacitated to connect with these services—including the running around and the paperwork.

Hopefully it won't be long before each county, city and state has a coordinator for benefits and services for the sick and dying.

SOCIAL SECURITY

Besides Social Security Retirement Benefits, Social Security administers five programs that may be useful to you and the dying person: Medicare, Disability Insurance, Dependent Benefits, Survivors Benefits, and Supplemental Security Income. They also determine eligibility for Medicaid in some cases.

The problem we encountered with Social Security was that their help did not arrive before Mary died. Hopefully you'll have more time, and they'll complete their processing in time to be fully useful. Ask about Presumptive Eligibility, which is designed to speed up the process.

Retirement Benefits. If you're 62 and not working and have paid enough into Social Security, you're eligible for monthly payments.

Medicare. If you're 65 and have paid enough into Social Security, you're eligible for Medicare. Medicare is a health insurance program similar to private health insurance. There's generally a deductible, and the policy pays a certain percentage over that deductible. Medicare can pay for *part-time* nursing, home health aide or medical social worker services, and for medical supplies and appliances prescribed by a doctor and furnished by a "certified home health care agency." If you already have Medicare, find a home nursing service that is certified by Medicare.

Disability Insurance Benefits. *Regardless of age,* if you're totally disabled and a doctor says you can't work for 12 months, or your disability is likely to result in death, you can receive monthly payments *if* you have paid enough into the system. Social Security requests reports from your doctor and determines if you are disabled.

You have to work under Social Security for 5 out of 10 years before you were disabled to be eligible. There is a five month waiting period where no disability benefits are paid. Payments start on the sixth month from the beginning of the disability.

Dependent Benefits. A spouse who is 62 or older, or people who have a disabled child in their care, or children under 16 may be eligible for payments.

Survivor Benefits. When a wage earner who has paid into Social Security dies, his or her survivors are eligible for:

1. A lump sum burial payment up to $255 payable only to a surviving spouse or a child entitled to monthly benefits.
2. Monthly payments — to a widow or widower 60 years old or if disabled at 50 years, divorced widow or widower married 10 years, minor child to 18 years, dependent parents, widow or widower caring for a child under 16 or disabled child (eligible for life is applied for before age 22).

Supplemental Security Income. This program is based on need, not on your having paid anything to the government. If you're 65, blind, or totally disabled, the government will supplement your monthly income to *bring it up* to $314 if you're single or to $472 for a couple (in 1984). This figure goes up every December. Your resources must not exceed $1500 if you're single or $2250 for a couple. They don't count the value of a house, the land it's on and a car. Most states supplement Supplemental Security Income and pay higher amounts.

MEDICAID

Medicaid is a state-administered health program for low income people based on need. Medicaid, unlike Medicare, pays nearly all medical expenses. There's no deductible. In some states you apply for Medicaid at your local welfare office, in others at a Social Security Administration office.

If you have questions about Medicaid call your state Welfare Department or Department of Human Resources. For questions about other federal programs, call your nearest Social Security Administration office. Much of your business can be completed by phone, and if you need to see them in person, ask which documents to bring so you don't waste a trip. If you're applying by phone, make a note of the date, who you talked with and the subject of the conversation in case you have to call again. To avoid a long wait, don't go in on a Monday, usually their busiest day.

VETERANS ADMINISTRATION

In your area there is a Veterans Service Bureau or Agency.

Any person who served in the U.S. Armed Forces with at least 90 days of wartime service and an honorable or general discharge, who's over 65 or totally and permanently disabled, is eligible for a pension. A single veteran can receive *up to* $459 per month, a married veteran $602 plus $78 a month for each dependent child. All your income is counted against the $459—they pay you the difference.

Depending on their income, a widow or dependent children of a veteran are eligible for a pension and educational benefits. If the death is "service-connected" (for example, if the veteran dies of an old wound, illness or condition acquired while in the service) there are additional benefits.

Eligible veterans who need help caring for themselves can receive an "aid-in-attendance allowance" up to $877 if married or $735 if single. "Housebound" veterans unable to leave home but who do not need other help are eligible for up to $561 a month if single and $711 if married.

If a veteran has to go to a private hospital in an emergency, the receiving physician must call a VA hospital within 72 hours and, if the veteran is eligible, the Veterans Administration will transfer him or her to a free VA hospital or will pick up the tab if she or he is too ill to be transferred. When a veteran dies in a VA hospital or while being transferred to one, VA will pay to transport the body to the home town or place of burial.

A veteran, his widow and any number of unmarried children under 18 can receive a plot and headstone free of charge in a National Cemetery. If a veteran who is receiving a pension or compensation for service connected disabilities is buried in a private cemetery, VA will pay up to $300 for burial and up to $150 for the plot and interment. If the death is "service-connected," there's a burial allowance up to $1,100. VA will also furnish headstones and a burial flag. Funeral directors have the applications for burial benefits and will complete them for you, or you may apply at the nearest VA office.

The VA doesn't chase you around the country to give you money. *You have to apply.* They have other benefits not mentioned here, and their laws and payments change often, so check with VA if you think there's any chance you or the dying person might qualify.

Legal Help

LEGAL AID SERVICES

These are government-funded, nonprofit services that can help with any type of legal problem including land transfers, wills and estate planning. There are certain income qualifications for receiving these no-cost services.

To find a legal aid service, look in the Yellow Pages under "Lawyers." For example, the service in Santa Fe is listed as Northern New Mexico Legal Services. If you can't find one in the phone book, call the county courthouse, bar association or lawyer referral service.

Note: Because of federal budget cuts these services may go out of business.

STATE BOARD OF HEALTH, MEDICAL EXAMINER, COUNTY CORONER

At some point you'll need to know about the laws in your

area regarding death at home and burial. This will enable you to plan a simple, dignified funeral that meets your needs and desires, and the *legal requirements.*

Look in the white pages of the phone book under the name of your state, county or city for the Board of Health, Medical Examiner or Coroner, or call your hospital or county courthouse and ask who to call. Funeral homes are not the best sources for this information because they have a vested interest in your spending as much money as possible.

Medical Supplies

RENTAL SERVICES

You can rent almost any of the supplies you'll need. First see if you can find them free of charge. If not, rent by the month, because the rates are less. For example, in our area you can rent a hospital bed for $45 a month, bedside commode for $13, and color TV for $35 with a $25 deposit. Look in the Yellow Pages under "Medical Supplies—Rental" or "Rental Services."

THE AMERICAN CANCER SOCIETY

This essentially volunteer group that works with cancer patients often provides free transportation to and from treatments or reimburses the family for gas. They may lend a variety of supplies: wheelchairs, hospital beds, commodes. They may also have dressing supplies. Some chapters will reimburse you for specific pain-relieving drugs. A San Antonio chapter has a caring service that provides disposable pads used for incontinent patients. Our Santa Fe chapter has a wig for someone who loses her hair from chemotherapy!

MEDICAL SUPPLY COMPANIES AND HOSPITAL PHARMACIES

If you're unable to find no-cost or rental supplies, check

with a medical supply company or a pharmacy near a hospital that specializes in selling supplies needed by patients at home.

Counseling

COUNSELORS

There are counselors who are specially trained to help us with our feelings. If this dying process brings up feelings which are difficult for you to deal with, consider getting outside help, such as a therapist, psychologist or social worker. It's a sign of courage, not cowardice, to seek help from a professional *if* problems seem beyond your capabilities at the moment.

You may already know people in your community who specialize in helping with emotional difficulties. It will be most helpful to find someone who is clear about his or her own feelings about death. Call a hospice for a recommendation. Check with a County Mental Health Association, Community Mental Health Clinic or a college. If you live in a city, look for a Council of Social Agencies or branch of the Family Services Association. For a child, you might check first with the school guidance counselor.

SHANTI NILAYA

The work of this center, founded by Dr. Elisabeth Kübler-Ross and infused with her love, helps people accept death as a part of life. *Shanti Nilaya* means "home of peace." Regular workshop-retreats are given for dying patients, their families and other care-givers such as nurses, doctors and clergy. A five day live-in retreat called "Life, Death and Transition" is given throughout the U.S. and abroad. These retreats are joyous celebrations of life in which you work with your feelings as well as listening to others. "Intensive Growth Psychodrama," a workshop to help people, dying or not, deal with emotional pain, is generally given at the center.

Dr. Kübler-Ross has written the following books which are useful in increasing our understanding of dying:

On Death and Dying
Questions and Answers on Death and Dying
Death, the Final Stage of Growth
To Live Until We Say Goodbye
Living with Death and Dying

She lectures in the U.S., Europe and Australia. If you have a chance to hear her, do. She's an inspiration. For her lecture schedule and workshop locations, send a self-addressed stamped envelope to the center. The center also has tapes available such as "Life, Death and Life after Death" and "Dr Kübler-Ross Talks to High School Students."

Shanti Nilaya
Star Route A—Box 28
Headwaters, Virginia 24442

THE CENTER FOR ATTITUDINAL HEALING

This joyful, loving group works with children and adults with life-threatening diseases. They use the principle "love is the only energy there is" from the *A Course in Miracles* books, which teach how to use love to transform the fear in our lives. Participants with life-threatening illnesses act as counselors for others with a similar challenge. Programs and support groups help young children, siblings, sons and daughters, adults and elders share their fears and anxieties and exchange loving support for one another.

The Center has a Phone Pal/Pen Pal Program to extend love and support with children and their parents across the country. It has books, pamphlets, cassettes and video tapes available. The children have created their own inspiring book, *There's a Rainbow Behind Every Dark Cloud,* which I recommend for any child facing a life-threatening disease.

The founder, Dr. Gerald Jampolsky, is the author of *Love is Letting Go of Fear.*

Out of compassion for parents already overburdened with medical expenses, they don't charge for the therapy and other activities provided. Centers are being formed in other cities; call to see if there's one near you.

The Center for Attitudinal Healing
19 Main Street
Tiburon, California 94920
(415) 435-5022

Spiritual Support

CHURCHES AND SYNAGOGUES

Your priest, minister, or rabbi will want to visit and share their compassion and services with you and the dying person. Calling one is clearly the choice of the dying person. Obviously the richness of your spiritual and religious life will support you as you face dying.

A priest can be called at any time to give the "Anointing of the Sick," a celebration of God's healing sacrament. It was previously called "last rites," and is given at any time to the sick, elderly or dying.

There are no deathbed sacraments in Judaism, although there is a tradition of *vidui,* a statement of confession as death approaches. This may be the recital of the *Shema* as an affirmation of faith or the traditional Prayer for the Dying. From ancient times, Jewish tradition has prescribed a mourning ritual which is compatible with modern understandings about the grieving process.

THE LIVING/DYING PROJECT

The Living/Dying Project offers a home-like living situation free of charge for those facing life-threatening illnesses who wish to investigate this process with compassion and consciousness. The director, Dale Borglum, teaches work-shops around the country, which may be arranged by writing to him at the Project.

The Living/Dying Project
P.O. Box 5564
Santa Fe, NM 87502

Emergency Support

FIRE DEPARTMENT - RESCUE SQUAD

These part-paid and part-volunteer groups may or may not be under the same department. They're close to my heart because they still seem to work on the principle of brotherly love. Without their help we couldn't have gotten Mary out of that second-story apartment! The fire chief in Santa Fe, who also heads the Rescue Squad, said, "If you need help, call us and we'll try."

A Rescue Squad can help stabilize someone for move-ment to a hospital, and is available for any life-saving activity. You may not need them for this but they're trained to solve unusual problems. For example, if you're alone—no neigh-bors are home—and a sick person falls out of bed and you need help to get them back in, you can call the Rescue Squad for help.

AMBULANCE SERVICE

In case you have to move someone who can't be moved by car, van or pickup, find out ahead of time about ambu-lance services and their costs. They generally require cash upon delivering the person. So be prepared.

He who binds to himself a joy
Does the winged life destroy;
But he who kisses the joy as it flies,
Lives in eternity's sunrise.

—William Blake
Notebook

Chapter 4

Getting on with it:
Preparations and Homecoming

Know that you are not alone.

Every heart in the world is part of every other heart. Even if there is no friend or family beside you, you are not alone. The energy that created and encompasses us is with us as we bring someone home to live until they die.

Strength beyond what you imagine is yours. Love protects and surrounds you as you meet each task of the day.

The everyday limits of time and space can be transformed into a sense of connectedness with all people. If you're feeling alone—as if it's all closing in or you just walked into a wall—close your eyes and imagine yourself part of a huge family that's experiencing the same things you are, even in the same moment. Think of the people before you who have experienced dying, family, friends, people you don't even know, and all of us who will experience it in the not so distant future.

Each heart in the world standing beside someone they love who is dying is connected with every other heart. *Two hundred thousand* members of our family die each day on our planet—one every 15 seconds in the U.S.

If you feel your heart is breaking, feel it breaking open. *Hearts don't break closed.* People close them. The courage or peace you may find in your Self is shared with us all.

Whenever you're troubled or don't know what to do next, *ask from the quietest, deepest place you can find in yourself*... and listen for the answer. Sooner or later you'll hear it. It will come with quiet reassurance. Trust what you hear. Your Self knows more than all those experts out there. *Allow* your sadness and fear, and know that you are more than these.

If you ask for help, it is given.

You cannot fail.

You are not alone.

What Do We Need?

Once you've decided this person you love will live and die at home, choose the room or rooms that are most comfortable and convenient. Consider how much the person can move about and the location of bathrooms. Is the old room still the favorite? Could you hear someone call from that room? If a room was shared, do the persons want to continue sharing it? Does the dying person like to be alone, or is a bed or couch in the living room, in the middle of the life-flow of the home, a desirable choice? Is there another place the family can be if the dying person wants to sleep or be alone? A cheerful, well-lighted bedroom not far from the main living space and kitchen is a possibility—or even a greenhouse or porch depending on the weather.

It's helpful to locate a bed so you have easy access on both sides. This makes moving and turning the person and changing sheets easier. Bedside tables are useful for bottles, tissues, medical supplies, flowers and other things you want handy.

Make a list of things you'll need and want and go about getting them. Look around for what you can find at home. A list might go like this (not all are necessary, not even the first):

1. a doctor (see the following section on finding a doctor).
2. prescribed medicines, particularly those for pain control.
3. a nurse.
4. a counselor.
5. a hospital bed—only if both patient and family decide it would be easier. It's not always necessary and can be upsetting to give up your own bed even if a hospital bed might be more comfortable.
6. a commode (potty chair), bedpan or urinal. Commodes have a plastic pan underneath that can be emptied. You can bring a bedpan or urinal home from the hospital or buy one. Urinals are only for men.
7. a wheelchair, walker, crutches—according to the patient's needs.
8. extra sheets and bedding. If you have a choice, choose designs and colors the person might like. Waterproof pads for beds and chairs. (Electric blankets are not recommended.)
9. extra nightgowns or pajamas that are easy to put on and take off. A nightshirt for a man might be easier than pajamas. If you sew, you could copy a hospital gown in pleasing fabrics and colors. Bed jackets or cardigan sweaters.
10. a glorious potted plant or bunches of wildflowers.
11. massage lotion. Try an herb or health food store for natural products.
12. a TV, radio, and/or a cassette player.
13. drinking straws that bend.
14. an extension on your telephone cord. It might be ideal to have two telephones, one near the person (on which you can turn off the bell), and one in a private place where you can talk and let out your feelings.
15. extra pillows.
16. alcohol, cotton balls. Hydrogen peroxide or swabs for care of the teeth.
17. a plastic dishpan for bathing.
18. paper towels and tissues. Also cotton towels.

19. socks and nonskid slippers. Feet tend to get cold if the weather is at all cool.
20. a stand-up bed tray if the person can feed him or herself.
21. two hot water bottles, one for the feet and one for easing pain.

Finding a Doctor

This may or may not be a challenge.

You need a doctor to give the patient and family assistance in making medical decisions, to prescribe medicines if necessary and to authorize nursing services, insurance benefits and hospice care. If the patient has to go into a hospital unexpectedly, a doctor can give directions that the patient's wishes in terms of treatment be respected. A doctor is useful for patient and family morale, although for day-to-day care a nurse may be more helpful.

You'll need a doctor who can understand the patient's desire to die at home and who is willing to support you. Try to find one who accepts death as part of life. If you're able, discuss with the doctor how he or she feels about death and artificial means of prolonging life and how the dying person feels about these things. This could save finding out later that the doctor you chose feels death is a personal or professional failure and will prolong a life no matter how inhumane this may be. When things are critical, there's no time for philosophical discussions. A doctor who's willing to work with you as an equal and be personally involved in this dying process will be the most useful. She or he needs to be available for home visits and phone consultations.

You may already have a doctor who fills the bill or you may have to do some looking. Friends may know of one; call a hospice, free clinic or university medical school. A growing number of young doctors are interested in home births and deaths. Call the local or county medical association and ask for a doctor who makes housecalls. Look in the yellow pages under "Physicians—General or Family Practice." Initial inquiries may be made by phone.

If the patient is taking medication, pain relievers, etc., make arrangements with your doctor and have them available before you bring the patient home. If you will be responsible for giving injections immediately upon the patient's homecoming, get instructions, syringes and needles beforehand.

Moving from Hospital to Home

When the patient is ready and things are sorted out at home, you're ready for the next part of the adventure. If you're nervous it's OK. At any time the patient, or the family at the patient's request, can check him or her out of the hospital. As mentioned earlier, it's easier if the doctor agrees and very uncommon for one to try to stop someone going home by instituting legal proceedings.

Driving a person home in your car saves the cost of an ambulance. Use a wheelchair if necessary to move the patient to and from the car. If an ambulance is needed, be prepared to pay cash. The doctor may ask a nurse or aide to call one or you can call.

The Homecoming

This may well be one of the most satisfying moments of the whole experience for you and the dying person. Homecomings with John, Mary and Dad were times of joy and quiet satisfaction. Don't be discouraged if there are snags or difficulties. You are both learning and adjusting.

If there are children in the family, they may want to make their own kind of homecoming celebration. Wonderful, as long as it's not too tiring for the homecomer! Joshua, Ben and I made signs to welcome Dad when he came home from his chemotherapy weeks; once we dressed as clowns.

You've already completed some of the hardest work, making the decision and getting organized at home. You and the dying person are doing what feels right and are taking responsibility for your lives. The house probably feels peaceful, purposeful, right. The homecomer is often content or joyful and relieved to be in familiar, beloved surroundings. Even if it isn't their own home, it feels like *a place for living*. The dying person regains more ability to have things his or her own way.

My own experience with homecoming has been one of *rightness* (not righteousness) in cooperating with life by taking responsibility for dying. My feeling of helplessness vanished, replaced by a new sense of purposefulness. *I'm doing what I want to do, being here for this person I love and it feels good*. A feeling like this can carry you a long way through whatever lies ahead.

Sit down and enjoy the satisfaction of your accomplishment and the beauty of home.

A human being is part of the whole, called by us the 'Universe,' a part limited in time and space. He experiences himself, his thoughts and feelings, as something separated from the rest—a kind of optical delusion of his consciousness. This delusion is a kind of prison for us, restricting us to our personal desires and to affection for a few persons nearest us. Our task must be to free ourselves from this prison by widening our circle of compassion to embrace all living creatures and the whole of nature in its beauty.

—Albert Einstein

Chapter 5

Medical Considerations

When to Call a Doctor or Nurse

You may find it surprising how little you need a doctor or nurse if you accept that the person you're caring for is dying. A doctor is properly called for counsel and assistance with some specific procedure, *not to make decisions for you.* Ask for help and guidance to make the dying process as comfortable as possible. Don't let their advice dominate the experience. Listen to doctors knowing they have information you need and also that their life investment is in hospitals and medicine.

Call a doctor or nurse if you feel you're in over your head. Call if you feel you don't have sufficient knowledge to take responsibility for a decision. Call if you don't know what to do and panic, and the panic doesn't subside. Call about pain, developing bedsores, catheter problems, constipation. Call if the patient wants you to call. If you can't reach a doctor, call a nurse. In terms of practical care, a nurse will often help you more than a doctor. A nurse can call the doctor and get orders for pain medication, etc. Much of what the medical profession can give is moral support.

There needs to be an **explicit agreement** about what the dying person wants the doctor to do. For example, a complication arises such as difficulty in breathing, perhaps due to pneumonia. Does the patient want to be rushed to the hospital, which may prolong the dying process? In times past pneumonia was called the "Old Man's Friend" because it can help a person to die. Is there a reason to cure it so the person can die later of cancer? There may be. The patient can always change the agreement whenever she or he chooses. In a dying process, the dying person may die at any time and there is no blame.

Working with a Doctor

Working with a doctor can teach us a lot about trusting and taking responsibility for ourselves and about how we deal with authority figures. Doctors are just ordinary people with a medical specialty. They have a difficult role in our society, indicated by their unusually high incidence of alcoholism, suicide, drug addiction and marital breakups.

We have set them up as gods, as knowers of mysteries we cannot hope to comprehend and we feel cheated and angry when they don't heal us. Perhaps this inability indicates the *source* of healing is somewhere else. It seems a little silly to make gods of specialists in livers or nostrils and sillier still to turn our lives over to them. After years of working with people who expect them to be gods, many doctors start to believe it themselves. Then, when a patient dies, they take it as a personal failure—and *we* also see it as their personal failure.

Until recently, most of us have wanted doctors to be in control of our health. So they've become habituated to being in charge and are astounded when someone wants to participate in his or her own health. A patient and family who want to are often labeled "difficult." I suggest it is better to be called "difficult" than to abdicate our responsibility which may later cause us needless suffering.

Patients and families have generally reacted to doctors the same way people do to other authority figures—with feelings of hostility and/or intimidation. Neither of these attitudes makes for an open, helpful relationship. In the long run it's not useful to have unrealistic expectations of doctors—expectations which prevent them from being who they can be—and it's not useful or accurate to assume, *The doctor knows and I don't.* The most beneficial relationship between doctor, patient and family might be a partnership of equals:

a. The family and patient see doctors as helpers, feel compassion for them and appreciate their expertise in an area (usually a limited one in terms of the total health picture).

b. Doctors share their compassion and expertise with the patient and family without suggesting they know it all and the family doesn't.

c. The patient and family take responsibility for themselves and don't expect doctors to make life decisions about any life except their own.

A doctor's life would be a lot easier if he or she didn't feel responsible for the life of each patient. When we feel responsible and things don't go as we'd like, we tend to feel guilty. A doctor can be *responsive to* and not *responsible for* a patient. Once we, as patients and families, get over the fright of not having someone else in charge, we'll feel a greater sense of responsibility for our own lives and increased confidence and dignity. A doctor's life might also be more meaningful if he or she were willing to be personally involved.

If during this dying process, you have a problem getting your doctor to answer your questions and hear your concerns, be very *direct.* Usually harassed and busy, doctors can seem like escape artists. You could say, "It appears you're telling me that you're too busy to talk now. I'd like to make an appointment to talk about John's treatment."

Here are three questions to keep in mind when you talk with a doctor:

1. Presently, in simple terms, what's going on?
2. What do you think is best to do from here?
3. How much of this treatment is to keep this patient alive and how much is helping make him or her comfortable?

After each question repeat back to the doctor what was said to make *sure* you understand and everyone knows you understand. Review the conversation. For example, "Did I understand correctly that you feel . . . such and such?" *There is no shame in asking until you understand.* Make notes if you have to. I write down medicines, then call a pharmacist or read about them in a standard drug book called the *Physician's Desk Reference.* (The "PDR" is easily obtainable by non-physicians—your doctor may give you last year's.)

If you sense your doctor feels death is a personal failure or a professional defeat and is resisting or obstructing the patient's right to die, you might discuss this feeling with him or her. Then, if she or he won't stop resisting the death, it may be time to get another doctor-helper. Get another doctor or nurse-helper if that's what the sick person wants.

Physical Pain and Pain Relievers

The most consistently voiced fear about dying and death is physical pain, particularly in the case of cancer. You may be relieved to know that advanced cancer is *not* necessarily painful. Some doctors estimate that 25 to 50 percent of advanced cancer patients experience no pain as a result of the cancer. For patients who are in pain, its management is important to enable them to live fully until they die.

Each of us reacts differently to pain because it is experienced by the *whole individual,* physically, emotionally, mentally and spiritually. So a unique pain relief program must be developed for each individual. With skilled help, we can control pain just as effectively at home as in a hospital.

Even as we move to relieve pain, we need to be aware of its purpose. Pain is neither good nor bad; it's simply a messenger that tells us something in our lives is not working or needs attention or that we're resisting what is happening. It's pain that moves us to leave behind old patterns and ways of being that no longer work. The more a dying person clings to the body, the more pain she or he experiences.

Perhaps the role of physical pain in the dying process is to loosen our attachment to our bodies and the illusion that we are our bodies. *"Hey, my body is getting uninhabitable. I need to consider getting out of here."* Notice there is an "I" apart from the body. Without a body there is no pain. **Death itself is painless.**

Dying people may be afraid to admit they're in pain, feeling ashamed to be "weak" or afraid of returning to the hospital. We can encourage them to speak up and not 'tough it out,' so they can use their energy to live well until they die. Having pain does not indicate weakness, just *humanness*. Suffering is not noble. Let the person know pain can be controlled at home so they needn't fear returning to a hospital. The dying person may also fear addiction. Reassure them that the therapeutic aim in their case is pain relief and addiction is not a concern.

Sudden unexpected pain, called *acute*, causes anxiety. Your attitude can do much to help the person experiencing it. Your fear and resistance to their pain increases their fear and resistance, and their fear and resistance increases their pain. So you can help by not saying for example, "Oh, pain, terrible. We've got to get rid of it right away!" Allow the person to learn what he or she can from it as you quietly move towards relieving it, if that's the person's choice. *Do what the patient wants. No human being should be degraded by having to beg for pain relief.*

You might try using the word "sensation" instead of "pain." Stephen Levine says in his book, *The Gradual Awakening,* "Taking the label off pain often changes the experience." Aspirin and different strengths of Tylenol can be used for non-severe *acute* pain. *If there is severe pain for which you are unprepared, call your doctor or nurse.*

Pain that endures over time is called *chronic*. **Chronic pain experienced by a dying person can generally be relieved.** Because we want to live until we die, it's important to know that alertness and relief of chronic pain can be balanced. To be conscious at death is a choice similar to being conscious for the labor of birth. Some women like to be unconscious and wake up with a baby beside them; others prefer to be awake, cooperating with and participating in the experience. Perhaps dying is the labor pain of the soul. Some may not care if they're unconscious and others prefer to be present for their dying. It's a personal choice. There's no right or wrong way.

Whatever the pain challenge, the patient and doctor should decide together which drug or combination of drugs might be most suitable. A pain reliever that works for one person may not work for another. A dosage therapeutic for one may be toxic for another. Consider drug allergies. (John Muir, for example, was allergic to opium and its derivatives, which include many commonly used narcotics.) A person may have to try a number of alternatives until pain relief and alertness are balanced. In the words of Ivan Illich, we don't want to turn "patients into pets," as many nursing homes do.

The secret of chronic pain relief is regularity. The pain reliever should be given at regular intervals *before* the pain begins again. Pain is much more difficult to control if it's very severe before medication is given. A skilled person needs to set up the time schedule which can, of course, be changed at any time to meet the patient's needs. Ask the patient to keep you advised of how she or he feels.

Recent studies and practice in many hospices indicate that *liquid morphine* is an effective pain reliever for terminal patients. Its chief advantage is that it can be self-administered. **The side effects of oral morphine and most narcotic pain relievers are nausea, constipation and sleepiness.** Nausea can be treated with anti-nausea agents such as Compazine, taken about a half hour before the pain reliever. Constipation can be remedied a number of ways (see page 112).

Narcotic Drugs Commonly Prescribed for Chronic Pain in Terminal Illnesses

Name	Relative Strength	Usual Dosages	Method of Administering
Codeine	1	30-60 mg.	oral
Percodan	2.5	1 tablet	oral
Talwin	5	50-100 mg.	oral, intramuscular, intravenous
Demerol	7.5	50-100 mg.	oral, intramuscular, intravenous
Morphine	10	10-15 mg.	oral, intramuscular, intravenous
Methadone	40	30-40 mg.	oral, intramuscular
Dilaudid	40	2-4 mg.	oral, intramuscular, intravenous

Commonly Used Medical Abbreviations

Abbreviation	Meaning
a.	before
a.c.	before food or meals
ad lib.	to the amount desired
b.i.d., b.d.	two times a day
b.i.n., b.n.	two times a night
b.m.r.	basal metabolism rate
b.p.	blood pressure
B.P.	British Pharmacopoeia
c., c̄.	with
e.g.	for example
ext.	extract
fl.	fluid
gtt(s).	a drop, drops
h., hr.	hour
h.s.	at bedtime
I.M.	intramuscular
I.V.	intravenous
noct.	at night
NPO	nothing by mouth
p.o.	give orally

Abbreviation	Meaning
p.r.n.	as needed
q.d.	every day
q.i.d.	four times a day
q.o.d.	every other day
Sx	symptoms
t.i.d.	three times a day
Tx	treatments
U.S.P.	U.S. Pharmacopoeia

During the first few days of taking a narcotic, a person may feel drowsy. As the body adjusts and the person catches up on sleep lost while in pain, she or he usually becomes alert again and may live fully the remaining time. If drowsiness continues, the dosage can be adjusted. The morphine solution is given every four hours around the clock. It may be possible to give a larger dosage before bedtime to eliminate waking a person (and yourself) in the middle of the night.

The morphine solution, called by hospices "MS" or "OMS," contains morphine, alcohol and cherry syrup. It's used instead of the "Brompton Cocktail" that originated in England which includes heroin and cocaine. MS or OMS may be mixed with juice, pina colada, Kahlua, Amaretto or any water-based liquid. For normal dosage, see the *Hospice Physician's Standing Order Form* on page 118. MS is dispensed with a prescription which must be renewed each time. So plan ahead. If the person can no longer swallow or is vomiting, injections or Numorphan suppositories may be substituted. Sometimes Prednisone (40 mg.) is given once a day in the morning to enhance the patient's appetite and sense of well-being.

There are many other effective pain relievers. Another useful combination is Dilaudid in tablets, changing to Methadone injections if the patient can't swallow tablets. (See the list of narcotic drugs commonly prescribed for chronic pain relief.) Narcotic actually means "sleep inducing."

Pay attention and stay flexible when using these drugs. For example, a doctor may say one shot should last five hours. The patient reports that it lasts only for three. Consult with the doctor about changing the dosage. Don't be overly concerned if a much larger dosage than the one listed is necessary for effective pain relief. Remember, my dad *started* with 12 mg. Dilaudid.

There are a number of alternatives to these drugs: Scotch, Bourbon or other strong spirits, biofeedback, laetrile, heat, massage, acupuncture, hypnosis, color therapy, LSD, Marijuana, Mescaline and laughing gas—or laughing. What is right for the patient is determined by his or her choice, influenced by the content and style of life before the illness.

Marijuana, Mescaline and LSD have been used experimentally with the dying process. The fear and hysteria built up around these drugs has obscured their useful medical qualities. The active ingredient of marijuana, THC, has proved effective in preventing nausea in chemotherapy patients. It acts as a mood elevator and tranquilizer, tends to retard weight loss by stimulating the appetite and potentiates pain medications so that less is needed. Mescaline and LSD, consciousness expanding drugs, seem to enlarge the framework in which a person experiences pain, changing the experience of it and sometimes eliminating pain entirely. Laura Huxley in *This Timeless Moment* describes the death of Aldous Huxley, an innovative adventurer in the human mind. Huxley used LSD in his last days in order to experience his death as fully as possible.

Stanislov Grof and a group at the Maryland Psychiatric Research Center, doing research with cancer and LSD, made an interesting pain discovery. Grof and Joan Halifax in their book, *Human Encounter with Death,* reported that pain is relieved by a "transpersonal experience" (a transcendent mystical experience in which one goes beyond the usual limits of personality and connects with some larger whole, perhaps God). See page 215 for one technique for guiding someone into a transcendent space *without* drugs.

The controversy involving laetrile, a substance made from apricot pits, as a cancer treatment is well known. The government dampened the controversy somewhat by reporting in 1981 that laetrile is of no value as a cancer cure. In my experience, laetrile did not cure John or Mary's cancer *but* neither suffered severe pain in the dying process. In Mary's case doctors were extremely surprised that she was not in pain. As far as I know, no one has studied the relationship between laetrile and pain reduction. Laetrile has been legalized in some states although it cannot be carried across state borders. You might want to check with a pharmacist to see if it's available in your state.

Breathing and visualization techniques can be very useful in working with pain. If there's delay in getting a pain reliever, you might try them. In some cases, they may preclude your needing drugs at all. Breathing can be as useful for dying as it is for birthing. When we feel pain, we tense up and tend to stop breathing fully. Our cells don't get the oxygen they need to clean out toxins and keep the nerve signals straight, and the pain gets worse.

So, one of the first things to do for pain is to **keep breathing.** Unless someone has had previous experience with breathing consciously, she or he may focus on the pain and fear and forget to breathe. As the helper, encourage the person to breathe deeply, to *breathe into* the area that hurts, and then down into the toes. Ask the person to relax, to "soften" around the area that hurts, and open him or herself to the sensation of pain. As the person surrenders, gives up resistance, more oxygen enters the area and the pain may lessen. The body senses that its message is received and relaxes. Keep repeating, "soften, relax, open."

Paying attention to pain helps relieve it if we don't judge it as bad! It just *is.*

I find it very helpful to combine breathing techniques with hot water bottles and foot massages. While the person is breathing into the area that hurts, partially fill two hot water bottles with hot, *not boiling*, water. Cover the bottles with a towel so you don't burn the person's skin and place them under the feet and on the area that hurts. If you don't have hot water bottles, put the person's feet into a bucket of medium-hot tap water. Put a hot washcloth on the forehead. Together these applications seem to keep energy moving throughout the body so the pain is lessened or eliminated. (Again, if the pain is severe and you're unprepared, call a doctor.) When it feels right to you, add a foot massage to further relax the person and to stimulate better circulation. Breathing and foot massages are useful techniques for calming *anyone* in a stressful situation.

Shots or Injections

There are two types (routes) of shots or injections used for giving pain relievers: **intravenous,** in which the solution is injected directly into a vein, and **intramuscular,** in which it's injected into muscle tissue. Intravenous shots should be given *only* by a qualified doctor, nurse or medic. If necessary, you can give intramuscular ones. Ask a doctor or nurse to show you how and practice ahead of time on an orange. The following instructions and diagram will help you as well.

Don't panic. Giving an intramuscular shot is not difficult or dangerous. Although giving a shot may be frightening to think about, you tend to forget your fear if someone you love is suffering in front of you. Remember, love transforms fear.

Have the prescribed drug(s) and the correct size syringes and needles available. If you've had experience in giving shots, you can protect a person's privacy by giving it in the arm or upper thigh. If you haven't, it's best to use the buttock.

PREPARING AND GIVING AN INTRAMUSCULAR INJECTION

1. Position the person comfortably to receive the injection and ask him or her to relax. If administering to the buttock, ask the person to turn the toes inward to relax the muscle. (The

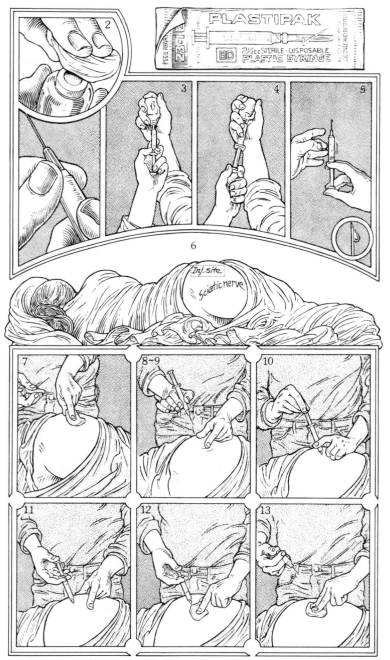

How to Give an Intramuscular Injection

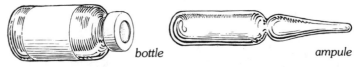

bottle   ampule

discomfort of intramuscular shots is usually due to tension in the muscle tissue.)

2. Swab the bottle top with alcohol. If you use an ampule, hold the top with a paper towel and break it off, holding the base firmly and snapping the top toward you.

   Remove the sterile syringe and needle from the package and check that the needle is secure. If the syringe and needle are separate, screw them together without touching the metal needle.

3. Insert the needle into the bottle or ampule. (*For a bottle only,* first inject air into it—the same amount as the dose of medication. If you want 1 cc. out of the bottle, inject 1 cc. of air into it first.)

4. Pull the plunger until the correct dosage is shown on the syringe scale and remove the needle from the bottle or ampule.

5. With needle end pointed up, tap the syringe with your finger and push in the plunger slightly to remove excess air. (Don't worry about injecting small air bubbles with an intramuscular injection. It may be uncomfortable, but isn't dangerous.) It's OK if a little of the solution spurts out of the needle.

6. Choose an injection site in the **upper outer quadrant** of either buttock (see diagram). This is important to avoid the sciatic nerve or a large blood vessel.

7. Thoroughly clean the injection site using a cotton ball saturated with alcohol or a prepared swab.

8. With the thumb and first fingers, press down, spreading the skin around the site.

9. Hold the syringe up and, like a dart, quickly and deliberately thrust the needle into the buttock at a 90 degree angle. (You'll find this doesn't rule out gentleness.)

10. With the needle in place, pull back the plunger slightly to see if any blood appears in the syringe. If it does, you've hit a vein and must remove the needle and choose a new site.

11. Inject the medicine slowly.
12. Quickly remove the needle, and then apply gentle pressure on the injection site with the cotton ball or prepared alcohol swab.
13. Massage the area gently and firmly to help the medicine be absorbed.
14. Destroy the used needle by bending and breaking it. (Some pharmacies sell a small, inexpensive needle disposer you may find handy if you have to give injections often.)

IVs and Dehydration

The question of intravenous feeding (through "IVs") may come up for you. IVs are used to nourish people who can't eat or drink enough to stay alive. The decision whether or not to use IVs in terminal care raises again the issue of the quality of life versus the quantity. Feeding the body cells by means of IVs often prolongs the life of the body. The cost is discomfort, less ability to move and the need to have a nurse. Dad said, "When I've got those tubes in I feel like a patient. When I don't, I feel like me."

The result of not taking enough fluids into the body is *dehydration*. The chemical imbalance created by lack of fluids often causes a person to have a sense of well-being or euphoria. It's a relatively comfortable death. The main discomfort, dryness of the mouth and thirst, is helped by sucking on ice chips and clean moist washcloths. It generally takes only a few days for a debilitated person to die from lack of fluids.

If someone has not yet accepted that she or he is dying and wants to be fed intravenously, a doctor or nurse can show you how IVs work and problems to watch for. There can be local pain and inflammation at the needle site. The needle can slip out of the vein causing the liquid to fill the surrounding tissue. A qualified nurse needs to be there or come by often to check the IV. Bottles are changed from three to six times a day. Don't worry if a bottle runs out. Air is not going to get in and kill the person. If the fluid is not running, a clot forms around the needle and the needle then has to be changed. Ask the nurse ahead of time what to do if the tubing falls out or comes apart or has air bubbles.

One of our worst fears about shots and IVs is that air will get in and kill the person. Actually, a surprisingly large amount of air has to go *directly into a vein or artery* before there's a problem.

Skin Care and Bedsores

Skin care is important medically as well as to help a person maintain dignity and comfort. If the skin is not properly cared for, bedsores can result. Bedsores (dicubitus ulcers) are caused when skin tissue breaks down. The first sign of skin breakdown is red sore areas. They occur where prolonged pressure limits circulation to the skin. Uncared for, they can become painful, oozing, raw areas where infection may set in. **The best thing to do about bedsores is to prevent their happening in the first place.** The less a person can move, the greater the chance of getting bedsores.

You can prevent them by *turning* a person in bed at least *every* couple of hours, *massaging* to keep blood circulating in the area, *drying* the skin well after bathing, and *exposing* the skin to air. Use a "sheepskin" (see page 152) under the person. Hospices often use eggcrate mattresses, foam pads with indentations like an egg box. They cost about $20 at a medical supply company and may not be necessary if the person is massaged and turned often.

If a person is so thin that his or her bones stick out, place soft cotton materials, like flannel, over the bones for protection. Cut a hole in a ½-inch or 1-inch thick piece of foam rubber and put it *around* the coccyx (tail bone) if this area is getting raw or painful. Place a soft cloth or pillow between the knees when someone is lying on his or her side and has been

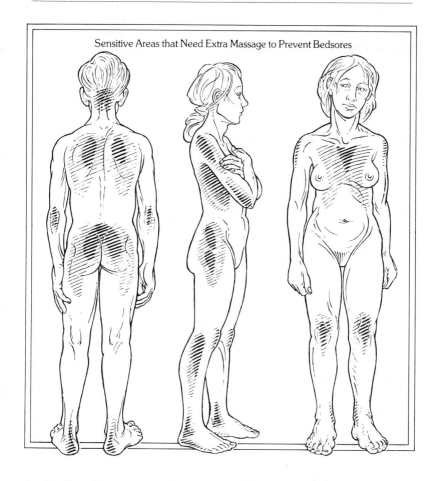

Sensitive Areas that Need Extra Massage to Prevent Bedsores

in bed a long time. Body surfaces that touch can cause pressure, friction and skin breakdown. You may also buy toughening cremes that contain tincture of Benzoin to protect the skin (Lanacane, Solarcain, etc.).

The basic idea is: if the skin is wet, dry it; if it's too dry, moisten it. Use a light skin oil like baby oil. Sometimes you're working with both wet and dry skin. Any areas particularly exposed to urine need to be washed and dried well. Use a drying cream such as Desitin, or powder such as Johnson's Baby Powder or Mexana.

If areas of the skin do redden or break down, **be sure to show the doctor or nurse and ask for suggestions.**

Elimination and Incontinence

Often a person who is very ill or very old will have problems with elimination. As diet changes and a person gets less exercise, organs are weakened and the bowels and bladder often start loosening or become blocked. Incontinence means loss of control of the bladder or bowels. Losing control over elimination, one of the most basic functions of our lives, can be very demoralizing. A person experiencing this loss needs our compassion and caring to adjust. See page 161 for ways to assist the person physically and emotionally.

CATHETERS

A catheter is a flexible tube inserted into the urethra (the canal that takes urine out of the body), and is usually connected to a plastic sack at the other end. It's used when bladder control is lost and can help prevent skin deterioration due to wetness. For men, there is a kind of catheter that is not inserted into the urethra but fits on the outside of the penis like a sheath. It's called a condom catheter. You'll need instructions from a nurse in the use and care of catheters and things to watch for, such as infection.

An alternative for dealing with lost bladder control is disposable cotton pads or diapers (see page 161).

Let the person know the alternatives and ask what they would prefer. Some people find catheters uncomfortable.

CONSTIPATION

A blockage in the bowels can cause discomfort and pain and eventually may be life threatening. **Paying attention to and treating constipation is an important part of home care,** particularly if your patient is taking pain relief drugs that cause constipation. A general rule of thumb is to use a laxative or enema if there has been no bowel movement for three days. *If there is undiagnosed abdominal pain, check with your doctor.*

Natural ways to deal with constipation are: activity; a diet adequate in fiber content; drinking warm water, coffee or some herbal teas; and using a toilet or potty chair instead of a bedpan. A diet containing bran, lots of fresh vegetables and fruits and their juices (prune and apple particularly) is helpful. White bread, white rice, meat and cheese tend to constipate. Acidophilus, a natural intestinal flora, helps relieve constipation and diarrhea by reestablishing the balance of intestinal bacteria—*very important* for people whose own intestinal bacteria have been killed by antibiotics or chemotherapy. It's available at health food stores in tablets or liquid form.

Temporary constipation may be relieved by a natural laxative such as Nature's Way or a bulk-forming laxative like Metamucil. For chronic constipation, you may use a combination of stool softener and bowel stimulant such as Peri-Colace or Senokot (no prescription required). If more stimulation is needed you can add Ducolax tablets or suppositories to the above. Some hospices use Colace, a stool softener, and 2 tablespoons of Milk of Magnesia before bedtime.

An enema is a simple procedure many of us have already used at some time in our lives for constipation. You can buy a disposable premixed one, such as Fleets Enema, or mix one yourself. Homemade ones are often more effective. Here's a recipe: Dissolve 2 or 3 tablespoons of honey or 1 tablespoon of castile soap with enough water to fill an enema bag, or fill the bag with coffee or comfrey tea (drinking strength). Place a disposable pad (see page 161) under the person. Put Vaseline or cream around the tip to be inserted into the rectum. Roll the person onto his or her **left** side and gently insert the tip three or four inches into the rectum. Hold the bag 18 to 24 inches above the person's hip and allow the water to flow *slowly* into the colon. Lowering the bag slows down the flow. Ask the person to breathe deeply and relax and to hold the solution as long as possible. When the person can no longer hold the solution and needs to evacuate, use a bedpan if going to a bathroom or potty chair is not possible. Be sure to wash and powder the area afterward, then wash your own hands.

If a patient fails to respond to a laxative or enema, a nurse or doctor will have to do a *digital de-impaction,* which means digging the stool out by hand with gloves on. An impaction is painful and unpleasant both before and during the digging out. It usually doesn't happen if you pay attention to constipation.

DIARRHEA

Diarrhea is the body's way of getting rid of something it doesn't want in a hurry. Unless it continues and/or the patient is getting weak from dehydration, it's often best to let it run its course. Cooked foods, including white rice, tend to slow down diarrhea as do bananas and Jello. Acidophilus will help rebalance the intestinal tract bacteria.

If these don't work, simple diarrhea is easily treated with medicine from the drug store such as Kaopectate and Pepto-Bismol. If it proves more difficult to treat, you'll need a doctor's prescription for Lomotil, paregoric, codeine, etc.

Sometimes a *little* diarrhea is a sign that stool is blocking the intestine. Liquid passes around the stool and it appears to be diarrhea. If a person's fluid intake and movement are limited, and/or they're taking narcotic drugs and the bowel has not moved normally, give an enema. Unless there is severe abdominal pain, it can't hurt and may clear the blockage.

Insomnia (sleeplessness)

The cares and concerns of a dying person may cause sleeplessness. If your patient has difficulty sleeping see if you can help without sleeping pills and barbituates. Addiction is not a real concern with the dying, but why interfere more with delicate body balances? Some possibilities are to take, before bedtime, calcium tablets (2 grams), camomile tea, valerian with B-vitamin complex, a warm glass of milk, or tryptophan (500mg.). Tryptophan is an amino acid in meat, milk and cheese. (Remember how tired you felt after Thanksgiving dinner?) Try a warm bath, hot foot bath, a back or foot massage, or a guided meditation (see page 215).

Stroke the hair and scalp and encourage the person to let all thoughts float away and let the head feel spacious and empty, clouds drifting in and out. When I can't sleep I use the Bach Flower Remedy, Sweet Chestnut (see Appendix B).

Avoid coffee, black tea and Coca Cola before bedtime. They contain caffein, a real eye-opener.

It's OK not to go to sleep even when someone else thinks it's time. Encourage the person to read, write, watch TV, listen to soothing music or think for a while. If not sleeping continues to trouble the *patient,* ask a doctor about sleeping medications. Hospices often use 15mg. Dalmane.

Fever

If the patient starts to run a fever, you can treat it with aspirin unless there is an allergic reaction to it. Tylenol is preferable if the stomach is upset or the patient has a problem with ulcers or bleeding. A tepid or lukewarm sponge bath can be very effective in reducing a child's fever. For a high fever, you can wrap a child or adult in cold wet sheets and cover them with blankets. If the fever continues or increases, you may want to call a doctor.

Depression

A dying person may experience depression. For the useful role it plays in the dying process, see page 123. Depression tends not to be as long lasting or severe at home, where the person has more control over life. If depression persists, the person may need help with counseling or mood-elevating drugs. I've yet to see *severe* depression at home.

Depression causes actual chemical changes in the body. Chronic pain wears us down until we feel depressed and hopeless. These feelings may lift when the pain is relieved, although some people become habituated to depression and it persists. To break the cycle, try to help the person refocus their energy. Because depression is often a result of not expressing what we feel, encourage the person to express sadness or whatever they're feeling and to live fully the time they have. Funny movies or stories may help. I also use Bach Flowers for depression (Appendix B). Some people may want to temporarily combine a pain reliever with an anti-depressant. Elavil, Sinequan and Ritalin are commonly prescribed anti-depressants.

Sometimes depression is a side effect of pain medications. Have your doctor change the pain medication or combine it with one of the anti-depressants mentioned above.

Irrationality

Irrationality is a temporary or permanent loss of connection with the generally accepted reality. You may not encounter it. I have only once, as a result of over-medication. If you do, attempt to find the *cause* or *unexpressed need* behind it. If possible, change the condition or meet the need.

Irrationality may be a result of pain, over-medication, exhaustion, blockage in the colon or emotional frustration. In these cases you can often reverse the cause. Sometimes it helps to change the person's physical position, for example, from lying in bed to sitting up in a wheelchair. Suggest a walk if it's possible.

Irrationality may not be reversible in the case of senility or a brain tumor. (Not all brain tumors cause irrationality. It depends on what part of the brain the tumor impinges.)

If a patient who can't walk tries to get out of bed, hold him or her gently and firmly, talk with them, massage them or whatever occurs to you to do. For their own protection, they may need to be physically restrained. You can use a restraining chair, a wheelchair with a tray that locks into place. If the person's in bed, fold a sheet until it's one foot wide, place it across the chest and arms and tuck it snugly under the mattress on both sides. Your doctor or nurse can also advise you about different types of restraints.

For severe agitation or hysteria, which I've not yet seen in my work with the dying, tranquillizing medication may be necessary. Haldol, Thorazine and Navane are commonly used. I regard them as a last resort when we've exhausted *every* other possibility. I would use them *only* to protect someone from harming themselves or others. Remember, we don't want to turn patients into pets.

If a person with a senile mind is sitting around not harming anyone and rambling to him or herself, the only change necessary may be in our attitude. Irrationality may serve a useful purpose in the dying process by allowing a person to disconnect from this reality and prepare for the next. If it's painful for you to witness, allow your sadness and remember that we all don't have to have the same reality, and we can respect another's reality. It can be interesting to enter the world of someone we've judged to be irrational and see what there is to learn.

Possibilities other than those I have discussed may arise and can also be taken care of at home. For example, if you need oxygen for the dying person, you can rent oxygen tanks. If the person is choking on secretions, you can rent a portable suction machine. A nurse can show you how to use these. Some other possibilities are included in the *Hospice Physician's Standing Order Form*. This form gives you an idea of what some care-givers do for their patients. You might want to share it with your doctor.

I encourage the use when possible of natural remedies in preference to synthetic drugs because undesirable side effects are minimized and delicate natural balances are often aided rather than destroyed.

DATE	O R D E R S
	1. Do Not resuscitate.
	2. Family conference as soon as poss.
	3. Social Service, P.T., O.T. to see pt. as needed.
	4. May have wine, beer, alcohol ad lib.
	5. DIET: as tol.
	6. ACTIVITY: as tol.
	7. SLEEP: Dalmane 15 mg (p.o.) @ h.s. p.r.n.
	8. DYSPNEA: O2 nasal cannula @ 2 L p.r.n. c̄ chronic lung disease.
	O2 nasal cannula @ 4-6 L p.r.n. s̄ chronic lung disease.
	9. COPIOUS SECRETIONS: Atropine 0.6-1.0 mg (IM) q.3-4h. p.r.n.
	10. COUGH: Tussend Expectorant 1 tsp. q.4h. p.r.n.
	11. NASAL CONGESTION: Sudafed 60 mg (p.o.) t.i.d. p.r.n.
	12. NAUSEA: Torecan 10 mg (p.o./IM/supp) q.3-4h. p.r.n. (if using consistently have Benadryl 50 mg (IM) available).
	Compazine 10 mg (p.o./IM/supp) q.4h. p.r.n.
	13. INDIGESTION: Maalox 30 cc (p.o.) p.r.n.
	14. ANXIETY: Vistaril 10-25 mg (p.o.) q.i.d. p.r.n.
	15. DEPRESSION: Elavil 25-50 mg (p.o.) h.s. or Sinequan 25-50 mg (p.o.) h.s.
	16. SEVERE AGITATION: Navane 2-4 mg (p.o./IM) q.4h. p.r.n.
	Thorazine 50 mg (IM) q.4h. p.r.n. or 25 mg (supp)
	Haldol 0.5-1.0 mg (p.o./IM) q.6-8h. p.r.n.
	17. ORAL CARE: Teeth cleaned, mouth washed, Vaseline to lips q.i.d., suction p.r.n.
	Artificial saliva 1-2 tsp (spray/swish/swallow) q.4h. p.r.n.
	18. EYE CARE: Isopto Tears p.r.n.
	19. ELIMINATION: Senokot 1 or 2 b.i.d.
	M.O.M. 30 cc h.s. or M.O.M. c̄ Cascara 30 cc h.s. p.r.n.
	Dulcoalx supp. 10 mg p.r.n. Fleet/K.Y./Oil retention/S.S. enema
	Lomotil 2.5 mg p̄ ea. loose stool up to 20 mg/d. p.r.n.

Hospice Physicians's Standing Order Form

-118-

DATE	O R D E R S
	Foley p.r.n. Replace q. month. Irrigate c̄ saline 2 x wk. p.r.n.
	Thorough peri care t.i.d.
	20. SKIN: Eggcrate mattress/flotation pad p.r.n. Observe skin carefully.
	Decubitus prevention measures.
	21. PAIN: MILD TO MODERATE CHRONIC PAIN:
	Oral Morphine Solution (O.M.S.) 5 mg q.4h. around the clock not p.r.n.
	Increase in 2.5-5 mg increments up to 25 mg. (if pt. is ↓100# use ½ as much
	O.M.S.). Add Aspirin 300 mg tab 2 q.3-4h. for bone pain.
	SEVERE CHRONIC PAIN:
	Oral Morphine Solution (O.M.S.) 25 mg q.4h. around the clock not p.r.n.
	Increase in 5 mg increments up to 40 mg q.4h. Then check c̄ physician.
	Use Numorphan supp 2½-10 mg q.3-4h. when no longer able to swallow or when
	vomiting.
	INTERMITTENT ACUTE PAIN:
	Tylenol tab 2 q.4h. p.r.n. or Aspirin 300 mg tab 2 q.4h.
	Tylenol #3-#4 tab 1 q.3-4h. p.r.n.
	Dilaudud 2-4 mg (p.o./SQ) q.2-4h. p.r.n.
	22. FEVER: >101° (R) Tylenol gr X (p.o./supp) q.4h. p.r.n. or Aspirin 600 mg.
	(p.o./supp) q.4h. p.r.n.
	John Bird M.D. 9/80

PRAYER FOR PEACE

(A version of the Prayer of St. Francis, used by Mother Teresa.)

Lord, make me a channel of your peace that
Where there is hatred, I may bring love
Where there is wrong, I may bring the spirit of forgiveness
Where there is discord, I may bring harmony
Where there is error, I may bring truth
Where there is doubt, I may bring faith
Where there is despair, I may bring hope
Where there are shadows, I may bring light
Where there is sadness, I may bring joy.

Lord, grant that I may seek rather to comfort
            than to be comforted;
To understand than to be understood
To love than to be loved
For it is by forgetting self that one finds
It is in forgiving that one is forgiven
It is by dying that one awakens to the eternal life.
            Amen

God bless you
M Teresa mc

Chapter 6

Being with Someone Who is Dying

Elisabeth Kübler-Ross' Stages of Dying

Elisabeth Kübler-Ross, a Swiss-born doctor, author and director of the Shanti Nilaya centers has served us all with great love. Her work with dying people and the attitude she brings to dying have given many the courage to look at a part of our lives that we've not faced before. Working with hundreds of patients, she noted a process that most go through as they die. Most people don't consciously want to die and this process is the way in which they make peace with this change.

The stages—*denial and isolation, anger, bargaining, depression,* and *acceptance*—are a **process,** not a goal. It's the same process many of us go through in facing any loss. Not all people go through all the stages; some skip stages and others move back and forth between them, sometimes from moment to moment.

The following description of the stages is just a clue to feelings you and the dying person may have. If our choice is to let people die in their own way, there's no need to push them through the stages to acceptance. *A person can die with dignity even if he or she never accepts dying.*

Denial and isolation. Dr. Kübler-Ross calls this the "No, not me" stage. It appears in the beginning of a life-threatening illness and often reappears many times. *"It can't be true."* The patient may shop around for different doctors or treatments. She or he may not want to "talk about it" or may want to be alone or with people who don't know what's happening. Shock, *numbness.* Dr. Kübler-Ross suggests that we just be there lovingly when a person is denying and let them know, *"When you want to talk I'm available."*

A person may need *denial* to cope with impending death, to adjust to losses already experienced and to tolerate the suffering or pain. Some die in denial—that's their way. As family and friends we may also experience denial and isolation. Check to see if the denial is yours or the dying person's.

Anger. The "Why me?" stage. Rage, envy, resentment. Anger at losing control. The anger is randomly projected, often on innocent people. *"You don't love me." "The doctors and nurses are incompetent." "Goddamn, God!"* Dr. Kübler-Ross suggests we not respond with nasty criticism or kill them with kindness. *Better to rub it in.* Affirm what's happening: "Doesn't it make you mad?" "Don't you feel like screaming?" The relief from venting anger may move the person toward greater acceptance of what is happening.

Sometimes the most loving thing we can do for a dying person (or people with a part of themselves dying) is to be a target for an outburst of anger. It's not hard to do if we **don't take it personally** and remember that expressing anger often helps a person accept dying. (I'm not suggesting you be a "patsy" for an angry bully, however.)

It's OK to feel scared if the person yells at you and it's OK to be angry with God. Imagining yourself in their place may help you understand. You'd be angry too!

Bargaining. The "Yes, me, but..." stage. *"It's OK for me to die if Eve and I can just take a trip to Hawaii first." "If I can just live 'til the kids graduate..." "If I live, I'll give my life to God."* Bargaining is a temporary truce. The patient may seem peaceful. It's a good time to take care of wills and other business. Dr. Kübler-Ross notes that very few people keep their bargains if they do live longer.

Depression. The "Yes, me" stage. Sadness. Dr. Kübler-Ross talks about two kinds of depression: *reactive,* for loss of job, a breast, the ability to take care of oneself; and *preparatory,* preparing for the loss of life and family. The dying person needs time to be alone during this stage to make the emotional preparations. This can be a good time for quiet hand holding.

Depression is the womb in which a new choice or way of being grows. It's caused by holding on to someone or something we can't have or by holding in some feeling we haven't expressed—anger, sadness, guilt, even love. Robert Waterman of the Southwestern College of Life Sciences in Santa Fe, calls one form of depression "trapped love." "We feel depressed when we block ourselves from *receiving* or *expressing* the living love that we are."

Depression is useful for a dying person and family holding on to a body. Making a change or letting go eventually becomes more desirable than the greyness of depression. You may be able to help someone see which feeling needs expressing.

Acceptance. "It's OK" stage. Quiet, at peace, neither depressed nor angry. Dr. Kübler Ross describes it as "time to contemplate the coming end with a certain degree of quiet expectation." The person is probably sleeping more; his or her concerns no longer relate to the outside world. It is "the final rest before a long journey." This period may be almost void of feeling. You can be there quietly, reassuringly. Again, resignation (giving up) is not the same as acceptance.

Our response to dying is like any other big decision we make in our lives. We can go from acceptance, having made a decision, back into bargaining or questioning that decision. It's very helpful to look for these stages in *ourselves* as well as in the dying person we love. It's important for the family to arrive at acceptance so the desire to prolong life doesn't contradict the patient's wish to die in peace. It's easier if we feel acceptance when we bring someone home, even if this feeling changes many times.

Telling Someone They May Die

I worried about this when I began to be with people who were dying. Like most of the things we worry about, it didn't materialize in any way I had imagined.

The first time I told someone she was dying, it was indirectly and accidentally. A nurse at the hospital asked me to talk to a patient with cancer who was dying and feeling depressed. I'll call her Rosa. I asked two nurses if Rosa *knew* she had cancer and was dying. Both said "yes." I talked with Rosa about her life and cancer and felt we had a beautiful visit. I left her feeling that communication had been opened and I'd be back to see her later. The next thing I learned, the head nurse and doctor were in a rage with some idiot in the Pastoral Care and Counseling department (me, as it turned out) and Rosa was furious! The doctor hadn't told her she had cancer or was dying. He felt she was too sick and would take the news badly. I got through all the anger directed at me without feeling terrible by remembering that I'd done what seemed appropriate at the time, and also that expressing anger would help Rosa accept dying. Unfortunately I was forbidden to see her again.

Generally the doctor will tell a person that she or he is dying. The doctor is the appropriate person to give a possible fatal diagnosis because he or she is *'believable''* on the subject of physical death.

Optimally, the doctor will have spent some time with the person and will be aware of how she or he is handling illness. The doctor may then sensitively give the person information about the disease and its possible or probable outcome *as the doctor sees it*. You can discuss with the doctor how this might be done best. It's *very important* that the doctor not take away all sense of hope. (See *Hope,* page 172.)

The doctor might say, "At this point your medical situation looks difficult. I don't know anything we can do medically to cure you, but we can make you comfortable. It's always possible that you'll have a remission or that a new treatment will become available." **Leave room for miracles.** They happen.

If the doctor is not straightforward with the person, you may want to talk to the doctor about it. If we *avoid* telling someone the facts, we're assuming responsibility for his or her life. **We can be responsive to another person and respect their rights; we cannot be responsible for them.** If a person wants to deny they're dying, that's their right. It's not our right, however, to take it upon ourselves to make that decision for them. If we don't tell someone, we are denying them the right to die in their own way. We are denying them the opportunity to get their affairs in order and to do things they've wanted to do, which might help them prepare for dying. We deny them the opportunity to try alternative treatments. *It's more stressful to wonder if you're dying than to know.*

Once a *possible* fatal diagnosis is given, there's no need to try to force someone to face it. Most people who want to know more ask questions. People who don't may want to pretend it's not happening. In one study, about 15 percent of the cancer patients surveyed did not want to know about a fatal diagnosis.

It may well happen that a person tells us he or she is dying and that we must prepare ourselves. Dr. Kübler-Ross says, "Everyone knows when they're going to die, although it may be subconsciously."

If it comes to you to tell someone they *may* be dying, you can do it only in your own way. You might ask, "How sick are you?" If the answer is, "Well, I'm very sick . . . or dying," you can say, "Yes, that's my impression too." Remember, you're not telling them it's the end. It can be a time of satisfying new growth. You might suggest that a very sick person ask *God* what's happening instead of a doctor.

If someone asks you what's happening and you answer honestly and without killing hope, communication remains open for sharing thoughts and feelings. A person may know she or he is dying and ask you only for confirmation. If you aren't honest this time, the person may not trust you or feel free to share with you in the future.

Being with Someone Who is Dying

How can we most usefully be with someone who is dying? Just by *being present with an open heart,* making space for what is happening.

An open heart is the most important thing we can share with anyone dying soon or dying later. An open heart is love without conditions and judgements. Not, "I love you if…" Just "I love you." No one is right or wrong. Fear, pain and suffering are not right or wrong. Dying is not good or bad. *Everything just is.* From an open heart we can sense all the needs of the person preparing for his or her great change. Listen, see and touch from "our" heart.

"Serving humanity," a phrase we hear a lot, is *recognizing our common divinity.* It doesn't necessarily mean being out there making the world over. Two people in a quiet bedroom can serve humanity. *We serve just by understanding that we're both individual expressions of the One.* We're not right or "up" because we're still healthy, and they're not *wrong* or "down" because they're sick and closer to dying. Just two people surrendering to life, to all the things you may have thought life was about and discover it isn't. And the challenge is: Can we keep our heart open to the other's pain and sadness without closing it and shutting off our own pain? All pain is everyone's. Can we be open to what the dying can teach us about life?

We serve by recognizing that *dying is OK.* If we resist a person's dying, we can increase their resistance. If we pretend circumstances are different from what they are—deny what's happening—the dying have to play a painful charade with us. *Pretending,* not communicating, isolates people from one another and makes dying very lonely for everyone involved. Pretending can leave you both with the "I-wish-

I'd hads: I-wish-I'd-said... I-wish-I'd-done..." Instead, we can do and say what's in our hearts. We can be open to this natural life process called dying.

The ultimate gift of love is letting someone die in their own way. Our work is to make a *supportive space* in which this process can happen. Let the dying person be where she or he is and don't try to push them to where *we'd* like them to be. They're not here to die our way but their *own* way. Dr. Kübler-Ross has said, "Dying with dignity is not necessarily dying with peace and acceptance, but dying in character."

Discuss all decisions relating to the dying person with him or her—even decisions about small things allow a person to maintain their sense of dignity and worth. *Help* people express their preferences. If someone is accustomed to saying "yes" to things she or he doesn't like or want to do, encourage them to say "no" to those things. You might want to practice this yourself. Rather than over-protect them, encourage a dying person to live each day fully. In the face of death, does it matter if someone dies a little sooner because they went fishing or to a concert or enjoyed a binge on lobster, chili or chocolate ice cream? (We've nothing to lose that we won't lose anyway.)

Don't assume that you know how someone feels—*ask*. Don't force someone to eat or smile or be social. Those may be *your* needs, not theirs. Try to be sensitive to their need to be with people or to be alone to adjust for the transition. Ask "Is there anything else I can do for you?" This may uncover a need you couldn't have dreamed of. Once when I asked my dad, he answered, "Just don't stop loving me or helping me like you are."

Albert Schweitzer said, "There is a modesty of soul which we must recognize, just as we do that of the body. The soul, too, has its clothing of which we must not deprive it, and no one has the right to say to another, because we belong to each other, as we do, I have a right to know all of your thoughts."

Conditioned by our cultural fear of death, people expect a

lot of difficult emotional and psychological problems around dying. In working with dying people and their families from many different backgrounds, I have seen few challenges the family couldn't handle. Those few related to guilt, which occurs less often at home than in a hospital setting.

So you don't sit around fearing "problems" that may never appear, here are some reassuring words from Dr. Sylvia A. Lack, from a paper she gave at the First National Training Conference for Physicians on The Psychosocial Care of the Dying Patient (what a mouthful!):

> There is far too much talk in death and dying circles in this country about psychological and emotional problems, and far too little about making the patient comfortable. Any group concerned with service to the dying should be talking about smoothing sheets, rubbing bottoms, relieving constipation, and sitting up at night. Counseling a person who is lying in a wet bed is ineffective... If people are cared for with common sense and basic professional skills, with detailed attention to self-evident problems and physical needs, the patients and families themselves cope with many of their emotional crises. Without pain, well nursed, with bowels controlled, mouth clean, and a caring friend available, the psychological problems fall into manageable perspective.

This is not to say challenges won't arise, just that you will be able to handle them.

Polite conventions and courteous fictions that people have maintained all their lives may drop away when they're dying. Old prejudices, resentments and grievances may surface; long-hidden preferences (as for one child over another) may no longer be glossed over. The dying person may pass through periods of generalized hostility to everyone. If you're the object of this kind of projection, know that *it doesn't matter.* You are who you are, not who someone else *wants* you to be or *imagines* you to be. Someone may insult an image they have of you, but that is not you. *You* are not someone's reaction to you. Instead of reacting to the reaction, you can choose compassion and try to look deeper—to the person's essence. Mother Teresa calls it "touching Christ in his distressing disguise." We don't have to like someone's personality just because they're dying. We can always love who they really are.

We also serve by respecting our own needs. With the discomforts of dying, a sick person may become demanding. If the person is being too demanding for you, tell them you can't handle it. We don't win prizes for being martyrs. If a person is acting irrational, don't be afraid to be firm. Again, look deeper and see what unexpressed need they may be trying to express, and see if you can meet it. There's no need to be *over-polite*—as when the dying person is afraid to ask for something or family members are afraid to do what comes naturally for fear of seeming pushy or hurting others' feelings.

Jealousy—feeling someone has something you don't— may come up. This is natural. Someone other than you may appear to be the special one. Look inside yourself ... how much more special can you be? You were *born* with your specialness. There will always be people who can see it and people who can't.

A dying person can also be a joy to be with. Take a moment before you enter their room to "breathe in calmness." *Soften. Relax. Open.* Be as natural as possible. Here is time you may not have made before for the quiet joy of sharing as a family, couple or friends. The illusion of time— that there are things to do, places to go—can drop away ... just moments for whatever *is!* Share your feelings and what's happening in *your* life. Ask the dying person's advice. His or her perspective from dying may be of great help to you.

When the person seems open, talk about what's happening, what they want done when they die, a will, what kind of burial ... Often it's evening or night when a person feels like talking. Listen and listen. If there are things you've wanted to say or talk about with them and haven't, use this opportunity. It will ease your grieving later.

People who are sleeping or appear to be unconscious can still hear you at some level. Say only what you would say if they were totally awake. People confined to bed do pick up the 'vibrations' of everything around them, perhaps more so than a physically active person who has more distractions.

Something I do each time before I go into the room of someone who is dying may be of use to you. I say a prayer that *God use me for whatever this person needs if that be for the highest good of us both.* Then I share my heart, sometimes with words or just with my eyes and hands.

It's a rare privilege to be with someone who is dying. I suggest you use this time to think about your own death, your own spiritual beliefs. As we accept someone else's dying we move toward accepting our own. See what you can learn from the dying that may be useful to you in your life. What is really meaningful in your life and what is it time to let go of? What do you want to be or do or say that you haven't? Make the most of the inevitable by *living fully each moment* and letting go of your sense of separateness.

If you find yourself working on two levels, one which says "dying is OK" and one which says "*their* dying is not OK," be gentle with yourself. They will come together. There's an old circus adage, "You can't learn balance until you've learned to lose it."

When we truly let go, the quality of death changes. It can become a "fresh breeze of God."

Trust yourself. Love yourself.

* * * * *

The Dying Person's Bill of Rights

This comes from the Southwestern Michigan Inservice Educational Council and appeared in Ann Landers' column. It indicates a growing concern among us about the rights of the dying. The bill shares the concerns of *some* dying people; more importantly it points toward the desire of the dying to choose what they want and don't want. For example, not all people want to die with someone present, but most want to make the choice.

I have the right to be treated as a living human being until I die.

I have the right to maintain a sense of hopefulness, however changing its focus may be.

I have the right to be cared for by those who can maintain a sense of hopefulness, however changing this might be.

I have the right to express my feelings and emotions about my approaching death, in my own way.

I have the right to participate in decisions concerning my case.

I have the right to expect continuing medical and nursing attention, even though "cure" goals must be changed to "comfort" goals.

I have the right not to die alone.

I have the right to be free of pain.

I have the right to have any questions answered honestly.

I have the right not to be deceived.

I have the right to have help from and for my family in accepting my death.

I have the right to die in peace and dignity.

I have the right to retain my individuality and not be judged for my decisions, which may be contrary to the beliefs of others.

I have the right to discuss and enlarge my religious and/or spiritual experiences, regardless of what they may mean to others.

I have the right to expect that the sanctity of the human body will be respected after death.

I have the right to be cared for by caring, sensitive, knowledgeable people who will attempt to understand my needs and will be able to gain some satisfaction in helping me face death.

* * * * *

Grieving

You can't prevent the birds of sadness from flying over your head, but you can prevent them from nesting in your hair. Chinese Proverb

Grieving is opening up to sadness or anger if we feel it, and releasing it. We *need* to grieve throughout this dying-living process to keep cleansing and clearing ourselves. If we don't we're liable to walk through the whole experience numb from the strain of holding our feelings in. When we become so full of sadness that we can't hold any more, we close our hearts. If we wait until "it's all over" to open the floodgates, the backed up emotion may seem overwhelming.

The gift of grieving is that it allows us to open to the great reservoir of sadness in each of us, much of it not even related to the dying process we're living now. Grieving is an opportunity to clean up old, old stuff, the 'attic' or 'basement' of our beings, so we can move ahead with greater lightness, space and freedom.

Let the person you're supporting, man or woman, know that crying is a way to cleanse ourselves so we can live more fully. Cry as much as you need, to give yourself more space for living.

You might want to take a moment to read Chapter 13, Grieving (page 241).

Pacing Yourself and Family Morale

Let there be spaces in your togetherness. And let the winds of the heavens dance between you.
—Kahlil Gibran

The time factor is often the great unknown in a dying process. Unlike a home birth, in which the baby is born within a relatively short time, a dying process has no fixed time limit. Not knowing "how long we have" is hard for the dying person and the family. For this reason pacing yourself is very important.

Nobody can face death all the time, neither the sick person nor the family. Unless you take time for yourself, for letting out your feelings and taking care of your health, you may well run out of fuel before the process is over. An early all out effort can exhaust you and cause you to resent the patient for taking so much of your time and energy. Contrary to all beliefs and appearances, you are not Superman or Wonder Woman, although a part of you may think you "should" be.

Before you get out of bed each day, you might want to ask yourself, "What nice thing can I do for myself today?" This might become a morning meditation in which you also focus on joy and love to give yourself more energy for the day. Meditation is not some mysterious Hindu or Buddhist practice, it means *living with awareness.* Being aware the toast is burning... being aware of God. Some people make it a sacred cow apart from everyday life. This is unnecessary. *All* of life can be a meditation.

Because you're probably spending more time at home than usual, use some of it to do things you've wanted to do and haven't. Pick flowers. Make a fresh juice cocktail. Take a walk. Write that letter. When Mary was with me I did a lot of sewing and caught up on paper work. Instead of thinking, *"God, I'm getting behind,"* I could think, *"Great! I'm getting stuff done I wouldn't if I weren't home so much."* While my dad was dying I continued to work on this book.

Eat as well as you can and get as much sleep as possible. Try to eat balanced meals and not live on coffee and doughnuts. Taking stress formula Vitamin B and/or brewer's yeast will help soothe your nerves and give you energy. If possible, keep your own bedroom. With Mary, I was comforted to have my own space—sleep in my own bedroom—and I could hear her if I kept my door open. If someone needs constant attention, you'll need people with whom you can rotate sleeping. If you have no help, you may have to sleep in the room with the dying person... and you may want to anyway.

There are endless ways of dealing with our feelings as they come up. You already have your own ways; see page 170 for others. *Remember, whatever your feelings, they're OK no matter how they feel or look to you.*

Taking care of family morale includes doing enjoyable things for yourself as well as with the dying person. Don't be afraid to ask for help so you can go out or have time alone. Go to the movies, dancing, bowling, hang out with friends and talk about it all. **You can be totally loving and not think about the dying person all the time.** Ask for help if you need someone simply to be with you. By asking, you give someone else a chance to share love. If they don't respond as you hope, respect their honesty. Perhaps they'll volunteer on another occasion.

The Quiet Mind (White Eagle Publishing Company) is a beautiful little book from England I've used for years to help me relax and sleep well. It's available through some metaphysical bookstores and Shanti Nilaya (see page 84 for the address). I also recommend Malcolm Muggeridge's book about Mother Teresa, *Something Beautiful for God.*

Sharing and Family Morale

Sharing with a dying person lets them know they still count. While you're emotionally letting them go, it's important for you to be conscious that they're not gone until they're gone.

What can you share? Share your feelings as it feels appropriate, but not to the point of burdening the dying person. It may be hard the first time—it gets easier.

Share time together. Share decisions. Share games. Are there TV programs or stories you can enjoy together? Read together. Remember good times together. Pray together.

What about asking the dying person to share the story of

his or her life or making a tape recording as we did with my dad? These memories may help the dying person understand the tapestry of his or her life, and be a source of joy and comfort to you.

You might want to ask yourself each morning, *"What nice thing can we do as a family or group of friends today?"*

See Appendix C for two games that may be fun to play with someone in bed whose mind is clear.

Visitors

The number of friends a dying person wants to see usually depends on his or her earlier lifestyle. People who like a lot of people around, like John did, probably will want to continue having people around. By contrast, someone more solitary, like Mary, probably will want to see only a few. Ask if it's OK for someone to bring a child.

Visits with a dying person should usually be short, unless the person indicates otherwise. Visits can use up a lot of energy and some people feel drained afterward. Feel free to ask if the dying person is tired and if, perhaps, the visit should end. If you or other family members want to visit together longer, move to another room.

Let visitors know what mood the person *seems* to be in today. If they haven't seen their friend for a long time, let them know how she or he looks now. It softens the shock if visitors know, for example, that their old robust 180-pound friend is down to 100 pounds.

If the dying person has expressed a wish not to see someone, don't violate this wish. I advise not sending anyone in who's extremely upset or full of negative energy. You might first help such visitors express their feelings with you. Then, if they have a real need to see the person, accompany them and stand by for the 'enough' signal from the patient. At the same time, don't overprotect. The dying person and visitor may have a misunderstanding and want to be alone to clear it up, which may make both of them feel better.

As a visitor, be sensitive to your friend, to what is appropriate to share with him or her now. Share love. Imagine yourself in his or her place. Imagine what it feels like if someone says, "You look great!" or "Let's go fishing next spring." What would it feel like to receive a get well card if you knew you were not going to get well? These are obvious clues to a dying person that someone can't handle their dying; they make real communication impossible. The dying person usually agrees to play along and pretend for the moment that the illness is temporary. If you're open to your own feelings, including sadness, your visit will likely give energy instead of take it.

If business considerations need to be discussed, first check with the family to find out when it might be appropriate. Instead of making general offers of help, such as, "Call if you need anything," make a specific offer: "I'll bring dinner tomorrow night" or "I'll take the kids to the zoo Saturday."

As people approach death, they need more and more time alone to prepare for the transition. Don't take it personally if the sick person doesn't want to see you or doesn't recognize you. This is not uncommon; there's no need to feel bad. Focusing inward and disconnecting from the outer world is a natural part of the dying process.

Children as Members of the Family

Allowing a child to participate at home in the death of someone she or he loves can be an incredible gift. Children can learn early that death is a natural part of life. Without automatically acquiring our culture's fear, a child chooses his or her *own* attitude about death. When a dying family member is isolated in a hospital, often with *"no visitors under 13,"* the child has no way of developing a healthy attitude. Even if our words say "death is OK," the child may feel something is wrong because she or he can't see or share in what's happening. Shielding children from death only makes its acceptance more difficult when they're adults.

The loss of someone a child loves is more bearable if she or he has shared in that person's dying process. The shock is less if the child has time to adjust gradually to the loss. Being at home together allows this gradual adjustment, as well as time for what can be a very beautiful sharing. A child's greatest fear is loss of a parent. At home together, the parents can help the child understand that in our hearts we never lose anyone. We feel sad that someone won't be with us and we can feel joy for the love we share that never dies. Since Dad died little Ben often comes up smiling and says, "You know, I can talk to Gramps in my heart."

The way to prepare children for the dying of someone they love is to let them know ahead of time about death. It's the responsibility of the family to talk about death clearly and truthfully when it comes up . . . even if it's hard to do. A good time may be when a pet or person they know dies. What a child imagines may be *worse* than the truth. Euphemisms and white lies mislead and confuse a child about what's happening. If you say that the person who died has "just gone to sleep," your child may be afraid to go to sleep. If you say that God took someone, your child may spend much of his or her life fearing or hating God.

Explain death in your own way. It may work for you to say that someone was too sick to get well and they stopped breathing; then go on to explain your spiritual beliefs. Reassure the child that she or he will get well from the flu or a cold or any familiar sickness.

Often children are afraid of the dark and of being alone and feel sad when people they love leave. It seems honest to reassure them (based on the experiences recorded by Dr. Raymond Moody in his book *Life After Life*) that there will be beautiful light, love and loving people to meet the dying person. See page 248 and Appendix H.

I might say, *"We're all born to learn certain things. When we've learned them we're welcomed home to God. All the people who love us who have gone home before, meet us when we come home. Like Grandma and Grandpa will meet*

Daddy. And home is incredibly beautiful with rainbows, light and love."

Dr. Kübler-Ross emphasizes telling children both sides of dying: the personal loss and that the person is going to a beautiful place. She says that we say, "Mommy is going to heaven," because it's true! If we don't share and explain our sadness about the loss, the child doesn't believe Mommy is going to a good place because there's no celebration. She also explains to children the idea of the cocoon and butterfly. We leave the old shell to become something more beautiful.

Children adjust easily to being around an adult or child who is dying *if* they are told what's happening. They adjust more easily than adults if they haven't been overly conditioned to think that death is terrible. They feel good about sharing the responsibility of making someone comfortable and will feel important to be included in this event in their family. Let them participate in any way they want. Ask for their help with tasks they can handle. Hugging, holding and cuddling are some of our best medicines for any age, and children are experts. If a child wants to stay home from school and help, and if this doesn't overburden you, consider occasionally letting him or her do so. A *very special school* is happening in your own home. Ben and Josh were a big help to us in terms of joy, humour and entertainment. According to the informative pamphlet, *About Dying,* other reactions of children to death may be:

> . . . anger at being abandoned, fear of having no one to take care of them, guilt that they may have caused the death to happen, and confusion about what happened. Help them express their feelings, fears, fantasies. Reassure them that death is not their fault, that they will be taken care of. Be patient if they bring up the subject of death again and again as they try to understand it.

Help children keep up with other relationships and continue to have friends in to play. Watching children quietly at play may entertain the dying person; if not, the children can be asked to play quietly in another room. To help them express their feelings, encourage children to say whatever they want to the dying person. Encourage drawing and telling stories. Stories children tell that don't correspond with an adult's reality are not necessarily lies. They're children's ways of sharing what they experience which can help us understand how to support them.

A wonderful gift for a small child could be a letter written by a dying father, mother, sister or brother, which she or he will understand later.

Dr. Kübler-Ross has written *A Letter to a Child with Cancer* (the Dougy Letter), a beautiful explanation of life and death that children can understand. It's available from Shanti Nilaya (see page 255).

Three other children's books I love that deal with the spiritual understanding of life and death are: Ethel Marbach's *The Cabbage Moth and the Shamrock* (Star and Elephant Books, Green Tiger Press, La Jolla, CA 92037), Marcus Bach's *I Monty* (available at bookstores and from A.R.E., P.O. Box 595, Virginia Beach, VA 23451), and Fynn's *Mister God, This is Anna,* for older children and adults (Ballantine Books).

ON CHILDREN

And a woman who held a babe against her bosom said,
Speak to us of children, and he said:
Your children are not your children.
They are the sons and daughters of Life's longing
for itself.
They come through you but not from you,
And though they are with you, yet they belong not
to you.
You may give them your love but not your thoughts
For they have their own thoughts.
You may house their bodies but not their souls,
For their souls dwell in the house of tomorrow,
which you cannot visit, not even in your dreams.

You may strive to be like them, but seek not to
* make them like you.*
For life goes not backwards nor tarries with yesterday.
You are the bows from which your children as living
* arrows are sent forth.*
The archer sees the mark upon the path of the infinite,
* and He bends you with His might that His arrows*
* may go swift and far.*
Let your bending in the archer's hand be for gladness;
For even as He loves the arrow that flies, so
He loves also the bow that is stable.

—Kahlil Gibran
The Prophet

Notes on Dying Children

I have not yet worked with children dying at home. Children are *people* as well as children, so much of the information in this book may help to support a dying child. I'd like to share a few ideas I've encountered during my work with adults that may be useful.

According to parents and other care-givers who work with dying children, children die more easily than adults. They have less fear of death because they haven't been as conditioned as adults have, and perhaps because they're closer to their source.

Dr. Kübler-Ross says a sick child's greatest fear is separation from Mommy and Daddy. There is less fear if they remain at home and if we help them understand we cannot be separate because we live in each others' hearts. Being home with a dying child, as with any dying person, gives people time to slowly come to terms with the loss and to share together as a family. I imagine feeling both sadness and a sense of satisfaction and peace when we have cared for a child ourselves and she or he dies quietly at home, perhaps in our arms, surrounded by love.

If a child must spend time in a hospital, I encourage you to be there. Most children are frightened of being alone in an unfamiliar place where unfamiliar things happen. Get permission from the doctor to stay and take turns sleeping in a chair or bed beside the child. This isn't always possible, so don't feel guilty if you can't be there. The nurses will do their best.

Dr. Kübler-Ross found that mutilation is another great fear of children. She suggests having a child practice giving shots or other procedures on stuffed animals to ease fear. She also suggests putting a big bed in the living room for the child so you can rest and cuddle or sleep together. There the child can live and be cared for in the middle of the family. Kids generally want to be like other kids. Within the limits created by the illness, help them to do this. Help them feel as happy and secure as possible by not overwhelming them with your grief. Again, hugging and holding are great healers for both of you.

For ways to deal with your grief see pages 132 and 241.

Dr. Kübler-Ross reports that even children three and four years old can talk about their death. It may be in a symbolic way. Again, encourage a child to draw pictures about what she or he is feeling. What the child draws in the upper left quadrant of the picture is believed to indicate his or her feeling about the future and dying. Encourage a child to talk about the drawings. "What's that about?"

Dr. Kübler-Ross deliberately "guesses wrong" a number of times about the meaning of something in the drawing. Then the child can hardly wait to blurt out his or her truth. For information about dying children's drawings, see Dr. Kübler-Ross's book, *Living with Death and Dying*.

Dr. Kübler-Ross sometimes talks with a dying child about death by explaining that God is a teacher, and she asks "Would God give you such a big job if he didn't love you and think you could handle it?"

We can also ask this of a child whose sister, brother, father, or other person close to them is dying. You can ask, "What do you think it would be like to die?" This may also be an opportunity to suggest to them that there will be light and love. Encourage an older child who is dying to write a letter to their mother and father or brothers and sisters.

If I had a dying child, I might turn to The Center for Attitudinal Healing and Shanti Nilaya for support (see pages 83 and 84). Both are *full of love*, have experience with children and have materials available. Through the Center for Attitudinal Healing your child can write to or talk by phone with other children who have the same challenge.

For most of us, accepting a child dying is even harder than accepting an adult dying. For a mother and father, it may be the hardest thing they will ever face. And there's no preparation other than living and loving fully each moment and holding our children lightly, knowing we don't own them. We feel children have everything to look forward to, everything in front of them. Perhaps it would help to remember that a child is complete and whole at each moment in the *process* of his or her life. Our vision might be more like the original Native Americans' vision. The following passage on "knowing how to die" is from an *Omni* magazine article titled *The American Indian Mind:*

> The distinction is often made between a linear or sequential arrangement of time common to Western peoples and a sense of the 'expanded present' common to Native Americans. Most native people did not understand their lives as a sequence of goals (getting an education, getting married, raising children, being an elder) at the end of which lay a sense of final completion. For them, once one entered adulthood, often at the age of only 10 or 12, life was complete. One could only continue to grow in that state—in the way a sphere, already complete, can continue to expand, to become fuller. There was no thought of not having done enough in one's life, of being too young to die, or of still having your whole life ahead of you.
>
> With that continuous sense of a full life, no one was tyrannized by the prospect of death. Any day, but especially one in which you were living to the hilt, was a good day to die.

I believe it's accurate to enlarge that understanding to include *all ages.* Everyone is complete at every moment. This doesn't eliminate the hurt, although it may take away some bitterness and resentment.

I'd like to share the story of one mother (who I'll call Sarah) that I feel points to a very important understanding.

Sarah had one child. Her life seemed to be going along smoothly enough, perhaps a little grey. Then there was an accident in the driveway; a truck backed over and killed her little boy.

I'd never met Sarah, but I'd heard bits of her story and wanted to ask her to read what I'd written in this book on children.

The day I phoned her was the ninth anniversary of the child's death! There was so much pain in her voice that I asked if she'd like me to come over. When I saw her, Sarah appeared as if the accident had happened yesterday . . . shocked, grief-stricken, eyes swollen, the curtains all drawn. She said that since he'd died she kept seeing the image of his mangled little body. She was living in hell.

I suggested we try to get in touch with the soul of the child and see if it could help her. Although this was a strange idea to her, she was in so much pain that she was willing to try anything. She lay down on the sofa and I "called in the Light" to help us (page 212). First I asked if she were willing to relive what happened before, during and after the accident. Reliving the experience was *extremely* painful. Then I asked if the soul of the child was willing to be present. It was.

Sarah began to talk with it, not in spoken words. The child's soul was enormously loving with her and told her it needed to be free. It was *caught* in the mangled image she carried and needed to get on with its life. I suggested she ask the soul why it had been born to her and lived so briefly.

The child answered, *"I chose out of love to be born into your life to teach you to love yourself."*

I asked, "Are you willing right now to give yourself the same love you've given to the child?" The moment she did, the room filled with light and the mangled image changed to an exquisite being of light. This being asked her to send love to herself and to see this image whenever she thought of the child.

When Sarah agreed, she was free. All the bitter aridness lifted. I was deeply moved and grateful to God.

Over a year later she was feeling fine about her boy and said, "A child is a sacred trust that can be removed at any time."

'Guiding' of this kind should be facilitated by a person with training—see page 215.

I'm beginning to see some threads in the pattern of children who live only a short time. I'd be grateful if you'd be willing to share with me what you learn from working with your child, whether or not it's similar to my understanding. What you find out may help another mother and father.

I believe there is so much love in each of us that we create a child partially as a place to put that love. Often we place all our love in the child and if she or he dies, we think love is gone. Perhaps a child dies to give us an opportunity to remember that **we are love,** and love is not just in the place we put it.

Besides coming to gain experience to be fully who he or she can be, perhaps each child comes to teach us love—that quality that allows us to experience that *life is sacred, your life and my life are sacred.* Are going to school, growing up or getting a job a greater purpose for life than teaching love? I believe there is no such thing as a 'child', only wise old souls in children's bodies.

The pain we feel when a child dies comes from holding on—not recognizing that our very nature is love—and believing that love ends when the object of our love changes form. The child was never really 'ours' to begin with. She or he always belonged to God.

Use this opportunity to give love to the child within you as well as the child outside. I believe loving ourselves is the greatest gift we can give to our children (physically present or not), to our families, to our friends and to God. When we love ourselves, we automatically love others.

Life is made sacred by your love.

You are love. You come from love. You are made by love. You cannot cease to be love.

The whole manifestation is the manifestation of love. God himself is love. So the love which comes from the source, returns to the Source—and the purpose of life is accomplished in this.

—Hazrat Inayat Khan
The Purpose of Life

Chapter 7

Making the Senses Comfortable – Practical Home Care

For in the dew of little things the heart finds its morning and is refreshed.
—Kahlil Gibran

Nothing is worth doing unless it's done with joy.
—a Fruit Deva

Caring for someone means making the senses of the body comfortable, as well as the feelings, mind and soul. A joyful, loving attitude as we provide physical care helps a dying person maintain or regain comfort and dignity. If we feel someone is glad to help us, we feel free to ask for what we want and need. On the other hand, if we feel we're a burden or nuisance, we're often afraid to ask. You might let the person know, "I enjoyed doing the backrub" or "Helping you is a pleasure, Dad."

I hope you're beginning to sense that this adventure you've begun can be a beautiful experience and even a creative art which you develop in your own way to please your patient and yourself. True creation comes from joy. Can you imagine duty creating a flower? Let yourself really enjoy creating comfort and beauty.

Dying well is a concern as old as we humans. What has changed is the meaning of 'well'. *Ars Moriendi* (Dying Arts), which taught the *art* of dying, was one of the world's first do-it-yourself books. In the 15th century, Caxton produced a book, *Art and Craft to Knowe ye Well to Dye,* which included instructions for everything from the art of blowing your nose to weeping well.

Part of making people feel comfortable is knowing what you're doing. I suggest tacking a schedule or list on the kitchen wall for anything you need to keep track of. The list could include times for medication, diet or who's going to be with the person if several people share the caring. Stay flexible, a list is just an aid. Remember, one of the reasons for being at home is doing what the dying person wants or needs instead of what's convenient for a hospital staff.

Touch

Your daily life is your temple and your religion.
—Kahlil Gibran

Touch is a way to share the love and caring in our hearts. It's important to all of us in endless ways, especially when we're dying. Touching is a way to express with the body that something beyond the body is important. A person is loved even if his or her body is no longer attractive or is even unpleasant to see.

In many slow deaths from cancer the body may become very unattractive physically. You may feel repulsed. It's a natural feeling. Keep your heart open and remember your touch is received by the person who owns the body. Neither John, Mary, nor my father had bodies of great beauty when they died, yet each was a person of great beauty. By touching a dying person freely and lovingly, we're saying, *"To me your body is not the only important thing about you."* This helps people understand that their bodies are only a *part* of who they are and helps them prepare to let go.

MASSAGE

Massage is a beautiful way to touch and make a person comfortable. It also goes a long way toward preventing bedsores. Even if you've never given a massage before, you can do it.

You may massage the head, hands, feet, back or whole body. Do what you have time for and feel comfortable with. I'm particularly fond of foot massages because it tires me too much to do a person's whole body. I often get the image of anointing the feet of Christ. The hands and feet both have nerve endings from all the organs in the body. By massaging them you stimulate and relax the whole body. (If you want to help a specific part, see Appendix D.) To avoid loosening possible blood clots, skip massaging the legs of people who have recently had surgery, have been bedridden for a long time or are elderly.

Here are some simple massage instructions:

1. Before you start make sure the room is warm enough and uncover only the part of the body you're going to massage.
2. Think about your love for the person.
3. Feel your hands as an extension of your heart and rub them together to make sure they're warm.
4. Let go of rushing around. Focus completely on this person.
5. Quietly enter the rhythm of their breathing. Align your breathing with theirs.
6. Gently place your hands on the person, knowing the flesh may be very tender.
7. **Trust your hands.** They may be uncertain at first, but soon your instincts will open to what feels good to both of you. Light flowing strokes can be very soothing.

8. Don't be afraid to ask, "Tell me what feels good and what doesn't."

9. If your hands feel heavy or cramped, gently take them off the person for a moment and shake them.

10. Pay particular attention to bony areas like the tailbone or shoulder blades. If they are white or reddened, use your finger tips and rub in small circles. This will increase the blood supply and help prevent bedsores.

11. When you're through, keep your hands quietly on the person for a moment, then lift them off very slowly and gently. (I say a little prayer to myself that God bless the person.)

12. If you remove your hands abruptly, the person is likely to feel a little deserted and shocked, negating some of the good feelings of the massage.

13. Cover the person when you finish and help them feel cozy. They may drift off into tranquil sleep or feel so secure and loved they want to talk about things unsaid before.

14. Wash your hands in cool water to clear energy you may have picked up.

You're probably feeling better now yourself. What we give to others is always for us as well.

HAIR

For many of us it's a treat to have someone comb and brush our hair, for others it's awful. Tangled hair can be uncomfortable, and who wants to look like a scarecrow? If visitors are coming most people will want to look their best. It's also very satisfying to have clean hair and a scalp that can breathe. If a person cannot care for his or her own hair, you can do it. Brushing and combing may be part of a morning bathing ritual or done any other time.

There are several alternatives for cleaning hair. Hospitals generally use "no rinse" shampoo...you pour a little on the hair, massage it in and then towel dry the hair. You can bring "no rinse" shampoo home from the hospital or buy it at a hospital pharmacy. At a regular drug store, you can buy shampoo that sprays on like a white powder, dries and you brush it out. If someone can sit *safely* in a shower stall, you can wash hair and bathe at the same time

You can also wash someone's hair in bed if you need to. Invent a system that works for you and the patient. Be well organized ahead of time because hair washing is very tiring for someone who is weak. You'll need a pan, towels, and plastic to keep the bedding dry.

If the person can't sit up, put pillows covered with a plastic trash bag and a towel under their neck. Check the water temperature. Then lean the head backward into a plastic pan to catch the water as you pour it through the hair. Gently towel the hair as dry as you can. If the weather is cold, use a hairdryer to prevent chilling.

If you can't or don't want to wash someone's hair yourself, you might ask a beautician who's been trained to work with people in bed. You can locate one through a hospital or visiting nurse association.

Note: Don't forget to cut the person's fingernails so they don't scratch themselves. Some people enjoy a manicure, fingernail polish or light makeup. A man may need help with shaving.

CHANGING SHEETS

An important part of touch is having clean fresh sheets. A rubberized flannel undersheet helps the bed stay clean. Consider bringing outdoor freshness in by hanging sheets outside to dry in the sun.

Change the sheets whenever they're dirty, wet, sweaty or the person wants them changed. This may be several times a day or once every two or three days. You may save some changes by keeping towels around in case your patient spits up. It is tiring for both of you to change linen very often.

If the person can't get out of bed, you'll have to change the sheets with them in bed. A visiting nurse can demonstrate how, or use these instructions:

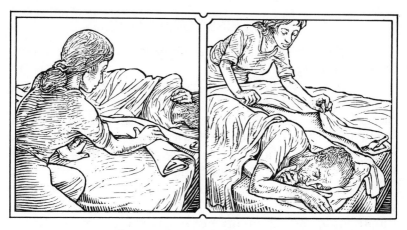

Changing sheets with a person in bed

Before any procedure directly involving your patient, explain what you plan to do and ask if it's OK. Have the clean linen handy before you begin.

1. Take off the top sheet and cover the person with a bathrobe or towel.

2. Roll the person onto his or her side with their back toward the center of the bed. Put the siderail up (on a hospital bed). Be careful the person doesn't slip off the edge.

3. Facing the backside of the patient, loosen the bottom sheet and roll it up until it's along his or her backside.

4. Position the clean bottom sheet on your side of the bed and tuck it in. Fold up the rest close to the rolled dirty sheet.

5. Help the person roll over both sheets to the side of the bed you've already fixed.

6. Move to the other side of the bed, pull away the dirty sheet and tuck in the clean one.

7. Change the pillow cases.

8. Help the person back to the middle of the bed and put on the top sheet and covers.

"SHEEPSKINS" AND PILLOWS

"Sheepskins" and pillows are important aids for comfort and preventing bedsores.

An artificial sheepskin is a washable synthetic pad about 3 ft. by 3 ft. You place it under a patient from shoulder to buttocks. They're available from a hospital supplier and some fabric stores, or bring them home from the hospital. (You've paid for them!) Have several on hand; one for the bed or a chair, another to exchange for a soiled one.

Have extra soft plump pillows available. For a change of position for a person lying on her back, place a pillow under the knees to prop them up. For a patient on his side, place a pillow between the knees so they don't get raw from rubbing together. If a pillow feels too bulky, use a soft flannel cloth. Tucking a pillow in behind the back feels cozy and prevents rolling.

You can also buy foam rubber wedges shaped like triangles. They're useful to position swollen ankles and calves to knee height, which alleviates some discomfort.

HUGGING, HOLDING AND CUDDLING

This is not the name of a law firm. They're a cure for loneliness and our illusion of separateness. As long as they come from unconditional love, I don't think we can over-hug or over-cuddle. Sharing love and warmth may include a person's sexuality. And this is OK.

Don't be afraid to ask for a hug. Your asking gives people a splendid opportunity, and if they don't want to give or share one they can always say 'no.' I suggest you call a morning 'hug time' for your family. It's a great way to start the day. Jog to a friend's house for a hug. I once started a 'morning hug' for my construction crew. We were the happiest workers on the site.

Your hugging, holding and cuddling with a dying person

obviously needs to be very gentle and appropriate to their needs.

Hug, hold and cuddle away!

Moving the Person

HOSPITAL BEDS

A hospital bed has some advantages for the comfort of the dying person as well as for the helpers. You can easily elevate the person's head or knees to change positions. The height of the bed is adjustable so that the person's feet may touch the floor when they sit up, which makes getting in and out of bed easier. The adjustable height also helps prevent back strain for the helpers because they don't need to bend down as far to assist the person. Transfers from bed to wheelchair are also easier because you can make the two surfaces the same height.

The disadvantages are that a rented bed is not the person's *own* bed and cuddling is more difficult. Giving up their own bed is hard for many people. We used hospital beds with John and Mary. When Dad was asked if he wanted one, he didn't even bother to reply. He wasn't about to give up the bed he had shared with Mom for the last 43 years.

If you reach a point when you feel a hospital bed would be less strain for you both, explain the advantages and ask delicately. Sometimes a little inconvenience is better than a change.

You can rent a hospital bed with electric or manual controls from a rental company. The manually operated ones are less expensive and perfectly adequate. On the other hand, some people love to push buttons and be able to change positions when they want to.

WHEELCHAIRS

A wheelchair gives a person who can't walk greater mobility and a change of scenery; finding one is easy. The American Cancer Society, some veterans organizations, and other service groups loan wheelchairs, and rental companies rent them at reasonable monthly rates.

There are a variety of models including one with a tray that locks in place if your patient's getting up and wandering around is a concern. If you have a choice, choose a model that most suits the needs of the person.

To prevent accidents make sure the brakes are on before helping someone move in or out of a wheelchair. See the illustrations for how to move a person from bed to wheelchair and back, or up and down a curb.

MOVING A PERSON WHO NEEDS HELP

During a home dying you'll have challenges helping the person in and out of bed, to a chair, to the bathroom or potty chair, etc. Be sensitive to how much help the person needs. *Overhelping* undermines a person's sense of worth and dignity. Encourage the person to help him or herself unless it's too difficult or too discouraging. Move them the way they want to be moved. Support them in places they can't support themselves.

A visiting nurse can most easily demonstrate methods of moving a person. I'll share some ways I use; you may invent your own.

It's important to learn how to do it with the least strain on yourself. One person can probably give all the support needed in the beginning. Later, you may need two. Some principles of healthy body mechanics when lifting and moving are: whenever possible, keep your back straight; use thigh and stomach muscles; bend your knees and keep your weight over them; take a wide stance with one leg in front of the other with your weight evenly distributed; hold the person close to your middle, your center of gravity. Don't lift a weight that you can slide.

To help someone out of bed. Imagine yourself in their

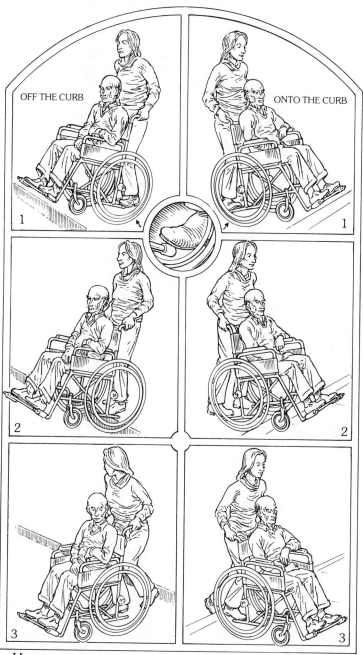

OFF THE CURB

ONTO THE CURB

1

1

2

2

3

3

How to get a person in a wheelchair up and down over a curb.

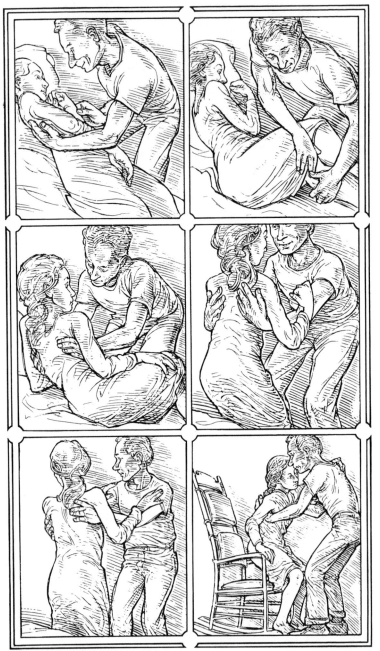

How to help a sick person from bed to chair. Awareness of balance and leverage is important.

place; sense what hurts and what's hardest for them about moving. Plan in advance *with* the person how you're going to lift or move them. What might get in your way? Any furniture or slippery rugs? Use non-skid slippers or bare feet.

If the person is moving to a chair or potty chair, place the chair at the side of the bed with its back facing the foot of the bed. When the person is ready to move, take a deep breath and relax yourself. Relax your knees. If the move is to a wheelchair, make sure the brake is on and arm or foot rests aren't in the way. Then:

1. Roll the person to her side, facing you. Drop the siderail if there is one.
2. Raise the head of a hospital bed.
3. Slide her legs partially over the side of the bed.
4. If she can't sit up alone, put one arm around the back of the shoulders, supporting the neck, and with the other arm gently pull her forward.
5. Stop a moment to let her get her balance sitting up. Make sure her feet are squarely in front of her.
6. If she can't help, face her, bend your knees and put both arms around her, under her arms like a big hug. I sometimes put a hand under one buttock.
7. Brace one of your knees against her knee to prevent falling if her knees buckle, and gently lift her up. (This is the waltz!)
8. Let her get her balance standing and, in this hugging "waltzing" position, move toward your destination.
9. If she doesn't need this much support, hold her under the armpits from the back.

To help a person in bed turn to their side. Raise the siderail (if any), place one hand on the far shoulder and the other on the far hip. With your feet apart, gently roll the person toward you. Most patients can help by grasping the siderail or bed edge on the side they're turning toward.

Moving someone up in bed (toward the head of the bed). This can be done by one person if the patient is light or can help. Two are necessary for a heavy person who can't. There are a number of possibilities:

1. If the person can help, have him bend his knees. Remove the pillows. Standing beside him, slide your arms under his back and thighs. Then, shift your weight forward toward the head of the bed as he pushes upward.
2. If the person can't help, use the same procedure as above, or two people can lift him with their arms under the head, shoulders and hips.
3. A *tug* or *draw sheet* is a doubled sheet placed under someone from neck to buttocks. It's used by two people to move someone up or down the bed. Place it between the bottom sheet and the sheepskin. Stand on opposite sides of the bed and roll the ends of the draw sheet toward the person in the center of the bed. Grip the rolled part firmly and lift-slide the person up or down. *Be sure to support the person's neck.*

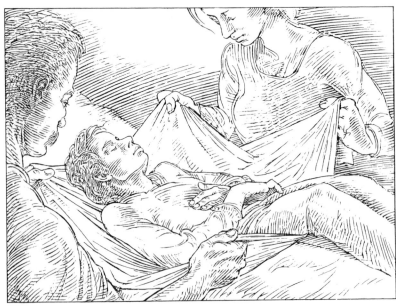

Moving a Person in Bed with a Draw Sheet

After moving someone, help make him or her comfortable. Rearrange pillows and the pad between the knees and straighten the gown or nightshirt.

Remember the Princess and the Pea? People in bed are often super-sensitive to things you might not notice or feel. Some little irritation may make a person feel crazy if they can't move enough to do anything about it. As death approaches you may have to move a person frequently. Trust your own loving tenderness. Relax and keep healthy body mechanics in mind so you don't strain your back. If you do (I have), don't be shy about asking someone for a massage.

Smell

What smells good when you're sick? Flowers, fresh air, sheets full of sunlight, incense, perfume? Ask your patient what smells she or he *doesn't* like. Perhaps the smell of food cooking is nauseating. Smell is more highly developed in some people than others, but most of us like to smell *good* and smell *good things. Good* is different for everyone! One character in the play, *The Mad Woman of Chaillot,* loves garbage because "it's the smell of God's plenty!" Smell has a lot to do with cleanliness.

Cleanliness

BATHING AND CHANGING

Regular bathing is important for the health and comfort of your patient. If someone can't bathe or shower, bathe them in bed. Is assisting the person to sit on a stool in the shower possible?

Generally morning is a good time for a bath, but ask. Make sure the room is warm enough so you don't have to deal with frostbite after the bath! Chilling can be a problem. I use a natural sponge or cotton washcloth and a plastic pan for water. Find out what water temperature the person likes. Soaps *without* lots of perfumes and additives cause fewer dry skin problems. Have soft towels handy to cover the part of the body you've already washed. Be sure to gently and thoroughly wash the genital area as odors tend to collect there. There's rarely a need to splash around so much water that towels are needed under the person, but use one next to the person to catch occasional drips.

After bathing, use a skin cream or lotion to prevent itchy skin. Alpha Keri is used by many hospitals and there are natural products available at health food stores. Using baby powder around the genitals may prevent rashes. After her bath I gave Mary a short foot massage with cedar oil to stimulate circulation in her body. (Cedar oil is used by some Native Americans for purification.) If the person has poor circulation and cold feet, put on socks or knitted slippers or use a heating pad or hot water bottle. Remember to test the temperature and frequently check the areas touched by the heating pad or bottle.

Change gowns or pajamas at bath time and whenever necessary, yet not so often that you tire the patient. Gowns that open in the back are easier to take off and put on. Ones that go over the head are a pain in *your* back when the patient can't easily sit up.

TEETH

Cleaning a person's mouth is important. It's just awful to go through the day with "bottom of the bird cage mouth." If toothpaste becomes too messy, you might change to hydrogen peroxide. If a person can't brush their own teeth, do it for them with peroxide on a toothbrush or Q-tip. Spongy swabs containing a special cleanser can be brought home from the hospital or bought from a hospital supply store or pharmacy.

Someone who wears dentures may want to continue using them. This is fine as long as they don't pose a danger. Consult a nurse or doctor.

ELIMINATION

We need to bring all the compassion and caring we have to help people adjust to losing control of elimination. They usually feel ashamed and embarrassed at losing control and needing help. You might point out that the situation could just as easily be the reverse; she or he could be helping you. Remind a mother or father of all the years they cleaned up their child. A cycle is completing itself, and we're reminded we're not just a body.

Use of a catheter is one way to handle loss of bladder control. Another is to place a disposable cotton pad under a person who has lost control of bladder, bowels or both. Chux or Curity Disposable Underpads are available at a drug store. For women you can use a thick sanitary pad for extra absorbency. Keep nightgowns or shirts out of the way and change the pads when necessary. After elimination, wash their skin thoroughly and use powder or drying creme to prevent irritation or skin breakdown.

Not all dying people lose control of their bladders or bowels. If they do, they're generally on a bland diet with few animal products so the smell isn't bad. If it makes you nauseous, put Tiger Balm or perfume under your nose and breathe through your mouth. Remember, this may be you later.

To the end, Mary and John were able to get to a toilet or potty chair. My dad used a bedpan once and lost control of his bowels once when he was drugged to heavily to wake up in the night.

As long as someone wants to and is able to get to the bathroom, I suggest supporting their desire by helping, even if you think using a bedpan or urinal might be easier for everyone.

BEDPANS

There are two kinds of bedpans. The flatter kind (called a fracture pan) is easier to push under the buttocks.

To use one, roll the person to his side, position the bedpan under the buttocks, then roll him back onto the pan. Or, with a more mobile person, ask her to lie on her back, bend her knees and bring her feet up as close to the buttocks as possible. Put one hand under her lower back and lift up as you place the bedpan under the buttocks with the other hand. Ask her to help, if possible, by pushing up the hips.

You can leave the room and ask to be called when they want to get off the pan. Flush the contents down the toilet.

Bedpans and plastic urinals for men are available from large pharmacies and medical supply companies.

Sight

BEAUTY

Beauty heals.

For a glimpse of the power of beauty, take a moment to remember how you've felt throughout your body when you've seen something you found incredibly beautiful.

Recent studies indicate that the pineal gland, whose function has not yet been scientifically determined, is stimulated by beauty.

In the past the person you're caring for may not have made much time or space in his or her life for beauty. You can help them open to an experience of themselves they may not have had before—so that in dying the adventure of life continues.

Imagine yourself in the place of the dying person. Try to experience his or her vision of beauty, then do what you can to fill the room or home with it. Each vision will be different. Beauty to someone may be the old stained hat he has worn for the last ten years. Hang it up where he can see it. It may be a painting or weaving or the way sunlight comes through an old lace curtain. If you have a choice, choose a room with windows so the dying can still experience the outer world, the sky, trees or the apartment next door. The sunlight that comes through the window will nourish body and soul.

Hang up beautiful old or new things, move furniture, add a lamp or a bird feeder. Gather wildflowers; go to a florist. Check first with the person you're caring for. Maybe beauty is leaving things just the way they are.

You might also suggest that the person spend time imagining things she or he finds beautiful.

COLOR

We're just beginning to realize again the effect color has on us human beings. Play with color: Ask the person which ones she or he likes. Dying people often prefer the *lightness* of colors to the deepness—a rose or peach instead of deep wine. For me, for example, dying with reddy-brown bedspreads would be torture. Keep color in mind when you gather sheets, pajamas, nightgowns, bedjackets and bedspreads.

If someone has a craving for a certain color, it means she or he has a need for it at some level of their being. To the extent you can, *meet the desire for a color as you would a craving for a certain food.*

Sunlight contains all the colors, which is one of the reasons it nourishes us. If we're experiencing perfect harmony we don't need more of one color than another. Most of us, though, at some level are trying to bring harmony to our lives and need specific colors. This is particularly true for people with dis-ease.

There are books about color and its relationship to different diseases and states of mind. Many don't agree on which color does what, so once again we have to trust ourselves and experiment. Two useful books are *Color and Music in the New Age* by Corinne Heline, and *Color Therapy* by Linda Clark.

Here are some general ideas to test. Greens through clear azure blues tend to be calming; yellows energize. Peachy pinks help those with emotional depression and people who tend to stay alone. (Some say peach is the color of love of humanity.) The range of orchids, lavenders and purples connect us to our spiritual nature. (Dad's favorite color when he was dying was purple.) Orchid relates to transcending matter. Some think cancer has to do both with deep grief —which is helped by the greens—and a lack of enthusiasm, which is helped by yellow, an emotional energizer. Orange vitalizes the body. If the dying person wants browns and grays, ask why. Those colors have to do with fear and pessimism, and your asking might bring up some unfinished business the person may want to talk about.

As you support this dying process, if *you* get a craving for a yellow dress or tie, treat yourself to it. There's usually enough money for what we really need and 'yellow' can be just as real a need as food or medicine.

TELEVISION

Lest I get carried away with beauty and color, we also look at TV with our eyes. There are some entertaining programs, especially on the Public Broadcasting System (PBS), that nourish the mind and spirit. Ask the dying person if he or she wants a TV in the room, and if so, when they want it turned on and off. If there's only one TV in the house, the person can still cooperate and sometimes watch someone else's favorite program.

Dad and I watched the world news together and with Mary I used to insist on seeing M.A.S.H. because it made me laugh.

If the sick person is interested in a particular program, this may provide time for you to be alone or do something else. A TV set with remote control, if affordable, might save running between rooms to change channels or turn it off.

Here's a visual idea from a friend: She prominently displayed a picture taken of her husband when he was healthy. When he was thin and gaunt and not so wonderful to look at, it was a reminder to everyone that he was still a human being who deserved love and consideration.

Hearing

SOUND

Sound has been used for soothing, purifying and healing since the beginning of humankind.

"In the beginning was the Word, and the Word was with God, and the Word was God" (John: 1). Does 'word' mean 'sound'? Perhaps *sound* is the One. Many people are just beginning to be aware of sound's role in the creation. At some level we've all been aware of using sound to heal: lullabies, Native American chants in the sweat lodge, Gregorian chants in the monastery, hymns in church. Sound and some kinds of music seem to clear our minds so new energies can come through us.

At home the dying person is blessed with not hearing doctors' beepers and clanging meal trays. Enjoy the sound of silence. Enjoy the sounds of home: birds singing, a child laughing, the same old leaky faucet.

Experiment with giving the gift of sound to the person you're caring for. Would a bell or a buzzer help a weak person call you more easily? Would hanging wind chimes outside the window be soothing? Some say chimes are the sound of the heart. They've been used for centuries in China and Japan. You can buy wind chimes at most import stores for $2 to $4.

MUSIC

What kind of music does the person like? Ask. It may be 'soul' or Beethoven's *Ninth Symphony*. What about flute music? Some say the sound of the flute is the sound of the soul. Pachelbel's *Canon in D* allows an opening to great peace without intruding. You may discover other 'immortal' pieces.

If you and the dying person have made music together, keep it up as long as you can.

Using the words appropriate for you, suggest that as the person listens to music he or she let go and *breathe in the music.* Tune into the harmonies. Music can be the needed break from the problems and routine of dying.

If someone seems to be holding in anger, one idea is to play a piece of music she or he doesn't like. It could help release blocked anger—and you'd have to be willing to take the consequences!

READING TO SOMEONE

Reading can be an enjoyable way to nourish the sense of hearing. Ask if the person would like to be read to. Reading can be a quiet, relaxing time for you both. When our attention is fixed and not wandering around among our everyday problems, other parts of ourselves may be set free. Being read to also helps someone keep his or her mind active and prevents boredom. It's not appropriate for everyone. Mary loved it. When I asked Dad if I could read him a book I love, Allen Boone's *Kinship with All Life,* he didn't even answer, which was an answer.

What about storytelling, prayer or meditation?

Often there is time for just talking together about the things we really care about, wonder about.

Be sensitive to noises that may be irritating or painful to the dying person (like banging doors, scraping furniture, vacuuming, etc.) Quiet for healing and final preparation is vital. Ask the person if there's too much noise or chatter.

Remember the sound of words of love. Use them generously.

Taste and Diet

Taste is a sense some will enjoy right until the end of this life, even when other bodily functions have closed down.

Once you've decided you're providing terminal care, trust the dying person to tell you what tastes good to him or her.

From my present vantage point, I'd ask for a little Cadbury's chocolate instead of mushed carrots. (This may change when my time comes!) During Mary's last week, for example, she twice craved butterscotch sundaes (or her memory of them) and we ran out to get them. She could take only a few bites and tended to spit them up, but she enjoyed the taste so it was worth the effort. My father wanted raspberry sherbert and grape popsicles. Conversely, if the sick person finds some food unpleasant, it probably means the body would have difficulty digesting it. If a person is indifferent to food, serve what's tolerable.

Before terminal care, diet is very important. There are different theories about purifying diets and which diet is most appropriate for which disease. You can find many books on diet in health food stores. Do as the patient and you decide is best. You can always change your minds. If you give the patient a certain food and later learn another would have been better, remember you did *what seemed best at the time.*

I suggest avoiding all artificial and chemically processed foods. When you're sick, you've enough to deal with without the weird chemicals the food industry uses for preservatives, coloring, etc. Fresh fruits, vegetables and grains are usually appealing and easy to digest. Try to avoid fried foods; they're hard to digest.

Chips of ice or iced drinks may reduce nausea. For a variety of flavors you can freeze fruit juices in ice cube trays. If chewing seems to be tiring, mash foods or put them through a blender.

If someone is on a liquid diet, make delicious and healthy combinations of fruit juices with yogurt, raw eggs or wheat germ and powdered vitamins. With a vegetable juicer, combine carrots, celery and spinach to balance the diet. Straight carrot juice is wonderful—if the liver is functioning well. Create and experiment. Use a beautiful glass and straws that bend to make drinking easier.

Remember those grim hospital meals wrapped in cellophane or metal on plastic trays? *Serve food as attractively as possible.* What about colored napkins, a child's cut-out, a tiny racing car or a flower on a food tray? For Mary I traded for beautiful plates with hand-painted rabbits and cats on them. Beauty and music can also soothe digestion.

Sick people often ask for a certain food and then can't eat it, perhaps because of nausea or blockage in the digestive tract. **If you're caring for someone who can't eat, their difficulty does not reflect negatively on your ability to nourish.** It just means that changes are taking place in the body. For a mother or wife accustomed to sharing love with food, watching someone she loves not eat can be *very hard.* (For my mom, Dad's not eating was the hardest part of caring for him.) The dying person can help by saying he feels loved even if he can't eat. Family members can help by suggesting other ways to share love, like massage or reading aloud, and by pointing out that her presence alone radiates love. *Dealing with a loved one who doesn't eat or eats very little is part of the process of letting go.*

Joy is prayer - Joy is strength - Joy is love - Joy is a net of love by which you can catch souls. God loves a cheerful giver. She gives most who gives with joy. The best way to show our gratitude to God and the people is to accept everything with joy. A joyful heart is the normal result of a heart burning with love. Never let anything so fill you with sorrow as to make you forget the joy of Christ Arisen. We all long for heaven where God is, but we have it in our power to be in heaven with Him at this very moment. But being happy with Him now means:

loving as He loves,
helping as He helps,
giving as He gives,
serving as He serves,
rescuing as He rescues,
being with Him twenty-four hours,
touching Him in his distressing disguise.

—Mother Teresa

Chapter 8

Living Fully with Dying — Our Feelings

As we come more into the understanding that working with the dying is a way of working on ourselves, we find that working on ourself means dying . . . letting go of the separate self, of every foothold and gesture that maintains our identity as apart from others and our original nature, our profound oneness with all that is.
—Stephen Levine

To live fully with dying we have to accept all of ourselves including all our feelings—the ones we like as well as the ones we don't. Each feeling is a teacher.

Take time to *feel* your feelings. This may sound silly but it's not. A lot of us ignore or run right over our feelings in the rush to *do* the next thing.

Our culture rewards us for *doing,* for achieving success, controlling nature, remaining young and thinking rationally. It's not often that we get pats for sitting quietly watching a stream, communing with God, listening to a child, being old or angry, or crying. We tend to forget the value of our feelings and of just *being* present now—this moment—for the child, stream or dying person in front of us. Then we're surprised when life feels meaningless or as if it's going too fast.

Supporting a home dying is an opportunity to slow down, to reappraise our values and to balance *doing* and *being*. And when they are balanced, life regains meaning, mystery and excitement. We then tap into a spring of limitless energy and have all the strength we need to support this dying person. Without the rest and nourishment of being, the constant activity of doing is exhausting. When we reach a balance, we rest as we go along and never have that deep tired-out feeling.

By helping the dying person understand that being is just as important as doing, we help them adjust to not *doing* all things they're accustomed to. If we primarily value doing, we can't accept death or help the dying person accept it. And dying is a return to our original nature, *being*.

Regaining this balance may shake up intellectual ideas and cause us to swing from one emotional peak to another. This is fine . . . part of the process of surrender. We swing until we regain our balance—perhaps until we make a friend of death.

As you support this dying accept the wisdom of your being; trust your feelings. After taking time to feel them, express them in a way that's appropriate for you. Once you've felt and expressed a feeling, send love to the part of you that feels it—your angry self, sad self, impatient one, lonely one, disgusted one, or the child in you. Then let go of it. If you have trouble letting go, try one or more of these: yell (possibly in a car), take a walk, jog outside or in place, take a deep breath, drink a glass of water. If you feel really scared or crazy, call a friend, counselor or whoever feels appropriate. Do whatever you can think of to release the feeling, then breathe in peace. Make time to reflect on what your feeling may have been trying to help you understand.

Remember, the dying person is not the only one under stress.

The following feelings aren't in a particular order. If you feel drawn to one, go ahead and read it now.

Hope

Hope is a reliance on the future that protects us from a "now" that is too painful. It's the question mark that is sometimes more desirable than an answer. As we walk through our darknesses, hope may help sustain us.

It plays an important and complex role in the dying process. Nearly all dying people have hope in varying degrees, although the focus changes. At first they hope to regain their health, then to live a little longer, then to die an easy death. Hope is useful to sustain them through suffering, endless tests and treatments, being in bed, and losing control.

Don't crush hope in the person you're caring for. He or she needs it until acceptance is reached. Hope gives time to come to terms with impending loss. It can be a sustainer and/or a form of denial. Whichever it is, we need is to support hope and be truthful at the same time. For example, "Your tests don't look good and it's possible the treatment will reverse this" (if that's true). We can always encourage someone to hope to live well until he or she dies.

The idea that there may be a cure around the corner, a new breakthrough in treatments, may help someone through a huge amount of discomfort. And breakthroughs are always possible. In the last couple of days before Dad died, he remembered with gratitude the doctor who gave him hope on the day, two years earlier, when he was first told he had cancer.

In her book, *On Death and Dying,* Dr. Kübler-Ross makes important observations about hope:

> The conflicts we have seen in regard to hope arose from two main sources. The first and most painful one was the conveyance of hopelessness either on the part of the staff [hospital] or family when the patient still needed hope. The second source of anguish came from the family's inability to accept a patient's final stage; they desperately clung to hope when the patient himself was ready to die and sensed the family's inability to accept this fact.

She also observed that in her experience, when patients expressed loss of hope, they died in a very short time.

Love

Our whole business this life is to restore to health the eye
of the heart whereby God may be seen.
                                                —St. Augustine

Love is the worker of miracles that restores health to the eye of the heart.

Just now, if you wish, take a few minutes to slowly read the following meditation. It is even more enjoyable if there's someone else at home who can read it to you. Use the meditation any time you need some extra love.

> *Remember some time in your life when you held and were held by someone you love, a child, a parent, a husband, a lover. Feel that again . . . remember how soft and open and full you felt . . . how safe and comfortable! Remember what your breathing was like and breathe that way now . . . feel the wholeness. Now give to yourself that love you were feeling with someone else. Give your love to yourself as you have given it to others . . . feel the fullness in your heart. There is a giver and receiver in each of us that keeps the circle of love flowing. We can give and receive love inside of ourselves, as we give and receive love outside with others. Feel yourself surrounded and enveloped by love. (It's there all the time whether we feel it or not.) Feel it giving you the strength you need for all the details, decisions and maybe crises involved with this dying process you're supporting. If you feel 'heavy' from worry, feel the heaviness lightening or lifting off.*

When we feel the love inside, instead of looking outside for someone to love us, our own loving abundance makes everything easier.

If you support this dying with love, you will likely experience that love transcends and transforms time. One of the reasons we love to love is because it moves us beyond the ordinary limits of time. Remember that sense of timelessness? The beauty and intensity of a relationship are often increased when one can see its end in time (death). Love, though, doesn't end with time; it belongs to eternity and dying is *leaving time for eternity.*

The presence of love gives the dying person a supportive place and time in which to experience the incredible changes taking place within him or herself. When we bring someone home we generally feel full of love; later, sometimes, it's difficult to maintain this feeling through tiredness, pressure or complications. Sustaining love is easier if we are aware of who we are and where love comes from.

I'll share with you my reality or vision of who we are to give you a context for understanding what I say about love and fear. If there is truth for you in my reality, or any other, it will resonate in your own heart.

In the beginning was God (unity, energy) and God was without form. For God to have form there must be duality—a positive and negative charge. So God created light and dark.* The passive dark had no need to express, but the active light did. So the part of God that wanted to express created humankind. The light is unconditional love; the dark is the space to receive it. When the light fills the darkness, there will be no more form. We return to God formless.

> *The formless Absolute is my Father, and God in form is my Mother.* —Kabir

Once we were created, we got attached to the form and forgot the formless. We forgot that God could not express without us. Fear was created when the first human beings judged that duality and separation are the same thing. Fear, the illusion that we're separate from that which created and encompasses us, prevents us from remembering we are God

---

* Other words for God are: The One, pure consciousness, The Word, Truth, Reality, Life, sound, spirit, the void, Father, Heaven, formlessness, eternity, infinity, Brahma, Tao, Dharma, Allah, The Great Spirit, The Kingdom, The Ultimate, the prime cause, the first mover, that which endures indefinitely. Some other words for light: The Light, Sun, The Son, Christ, Christ consciousness, universal intelligence, the life force, The Holy Grail, giver, and yang. For the dark: form, creation, earth, Earth Mother, the manifestation, the expression, Darkness, receiver, and yin.

and love in form. When we remember, we experience no separation between God in form and God formless. We are both.

So life and death to me are a process of remembering we are God and love. Sharing in the dying of someone we love can accelerate our remembering. (We've cheerfully acknowledged the devil in ourselves, maybe now it's time to just as readily acknowledge the god in ourselves.)

But if love underlies all of existence, why do I see cruelty, hate, greed, violence, guilt and insensitivity all around me? Why do love and fear seem to go together? How come I'm afraid to love? How come I'm afraid to receive love? Why am I afraid when I do love someone—afraid I'll be hurt, afraid he'll leave me for another woman, be in an accident... or die? Why do I see unhappiness in my relationships and in those around me?

Because, after we were created we judged we were separate from love, felt afraid and loved conditionally. "I'll love you if... if you remember my birthday... if you cut your hair the right length... if you have the right color skin... if you have the job I think you should have... if you'll never leave me... if...."

Unconditional love eliminates fear. Love is the *absence* of fear. Just, *I love you.* "I love you whoever you are... whatever you do... even if you leave me... even if you die. I love you without conditions and without expectations of anything."

Fear holds love a prisoner in the solar plexus where it's a possessive feeling. When we dissolve fear by loving unconditionally, love moves up and opens the heart. When our hearts are open, we experience everything as love; there is nothing other. *We've remembered who we are* We know love is the *quality* of our being and we experience God.

When we love unconditionally, we take responsibility for our love. It's no longer dependent on someone else—their presence, what they're doing or what they might think about our loving them. *When we take responsibility for our love, love connects us to joy, not to sadness and pain.* And when someone we love is dying, we don't feel like we're losing our love.

We love by loving, not by talking about it or preaching. When we love the person we're caring for unconditionally ("*I love you . . . even if you're denying that you are dying . . . even if you're afraid . . . or angry . . . or cranky*"), we simultaneously love ourselves without conditions. While loving others opens our hearts, to keep them open we have to love ourselves.

A common misunderstanding about love is that the heart is a container with a certain amount of love in it and we can give only that amount. This is the idea of scarcity. The heart isn't a container; it's more like a *funnel* that draws from limitless love. We can give more than we think we have and never run out. There's abundance, not scarcity.

Cruelty, greed, hate, violence and guilt are fear's distortions of love, and so are healed by love. People like Mother Teresa show us it is possible. My experience with dying patients and women prisoners has taught me that *unconditional love is the only thing that truly heals*. When we love this way, we recognize who someone really is, beyond the set of beliefs and concepts they represent themselves to be. *This heals.*

One of endless examples of the healing quality of love involved a young man with liver complications whom I visited only once. After 56 days in the hospital, no one could understand why he wouldn't let go and die. From his mother I gathered he hated himself because he'd been an alcoholic, had lost his job, and his wife and children had left him. I shared my beliefs with him—that I felt the purpose of a life-threatening disease is to help us remember who we are, Love; that he was not the personality he manifested as a result of a malfunctioning liver. I told him that at the deep level where all of us are one, I loved him. He died two hours later. The purpose of words is to love, to heal and to serve. *If you love somebody, tell them.*

Once we remember we are love, we're responsible for living that truth in our daily lives by loving unconditionally.

Don't feel badly or judge yourself if you don't do it all the time. We each love in the ways we're able to at each moment ... we're exactly perfect in every moment and we can be open to change.

> We are love not because we love, but we love because
> We Are Love. (after Schuon)

> Love is the Nature of God. He can do nothing other.
> Thus, to be God, love at each moment.
> —Angelus Silesius

The great gift the dying give us is the opportunity to remember we are love—the same gift we can give to them.

Compassion

Unlike charity, which has taken on the connotation of doing something for someone to absolve a sense of guilt, compassion comes from putting ourselves in the other's place and knowing, 'There by the grace of God go I.' Unlike pity, which belittles both giver and receiver, compassion makes us both stronger.

When you're with someone who's dying, it helps you both if you imagine yourself in the dying person's place. *The more we enter the world of the dying, the better we serve them and the more we learn.* We're better able to understand a need for help for dry lips, a need to talk or to be alone, even a need that may seem ridiculous to us. We learn more about our own inevitable death, and although this may bring up our fears, in the long run it will ease our fear of dying.

Love and compassion will get you through unpleasant tasks like cleaning up if the person is throwing up or has lost control of their bowels. *"I could be out of control like this and know that someone has to clean up after me."* In the process of putting ourselves in the other's place, we're cleaning up our own life (and death) because we're not so likely to see ourselves as separate.

Remember compassion for yourself. You deserve loving kindness as much as the dying person does. We often remember compassion for others while forgetting we're due it as well. People often feel unworthy or think that's being selfish. It's not. We can be truly compassionate with another only when we're compassionate with ourselves.

Faith

What is faith? Unquestioning surrender to God's will.
—Swami Ramdas

Faith is the belief of the heart in that knowledge which comes from the Unseen.
—Muhammad B. Khafif

For me, faith is trust in Life (unity, God)—moment to moment. It's trust that whatever happens is part of an orderly harmony of all that is. It's the *knowing* of the heart that transcends the *thinking* of the mind. The province of the mind is *time;* the province of the heart is *eternity.* To have faith we need the larger vision. Religious faith or beliefs may or may not play a part.

Faith allows us to feel peace and joy, even when we cannot understand what's happening in our lives. What appears to be separation, confusion or chaos is transformed in the light of unity and perfection. We all have faith to some degree or we'd stay awake at night worrying if the sun will rise again. So it seems that faith alleviates fear and gives us more freedom to live fully.

Because faith is a knowing of the heart and we can't 'know' in someone else's heart, it's useless to try to convince others to believe exactly as we do. Although we can share our experience, only their own experience can really convince them. Respect the faith of the dying even if it's unlike your own. Dying people quite often have visions or revelations that give them new or renewed faith that sustains them through the process of leaving the body (see page 247).

A person who has little faith is no worse or better than one who has lots. All of us have different ways of learning. Doubt and cynicism are valid ways to learn discrimination. Discrimination may in the long run be the ability to look so deeply into things that one eventually sees unity in everything.

Generally people who have chosen a rational/intellectual lens through which to see the world or who think being in control is the most important factor in life, find surrender (giving up control) very frightening. At one time or another, and that may be at death, everyone learns surrender. Once we surrender and see that the sky hasn't fallen in, we may *choose* surrender again. Then surrender becomes an act of faith, not just hollering 'Uncle' because the pain was too great. Doubters and cynics gain faith from their own experience, not by accepting what someone else says they ought to believe.

So we have faith by *choosing* faith—and rechoosing it and rechoosing it. Each day, each moment, we have an opportunity to choose faith in unity or to choose to see separation. If the doubter in us comes up and says, "There may be no tomorrow," we can thank it for expressing its reality and, if we want to, rechoose faith.

Faith that dying is part of the breathing in and out of the universe, and not an end, facilitates the dying process. Dying is more easily accepted by a person who feels a sunset is not the end of the sun and shedding a body is not the end of life. She or he will likely pass more quickly through the stages of dying—not skipping fear or anger but spending less time with them. Likewise, your work with a dying person is easier if you trust the *rightness of the process.* If you both have faith, dying can be a beautiful adventure into the little-known.

Joy
Joy is the essence of our being
The light that shines through us
The stars of our own recognition.
It's the sun in our heart that reminds us
*   Life is as divine on earth as it is in heaven.*

It's a candle that lights the darkness.
It's given us to remind us
Who we were before we were born.
The gift is always present.
It only waits for us to know its presence.

I remember joy in seeing a shaft of light in a stairwell, being tucked in bed, loving someone and discovering they loved me, finding a solution to a tough problem, greeting my father home from the war, playing with seaweed, walking barefoot on dirt roads . . . and caring for my friends and father when they were dying.

Others may remember joy in playing in water bursting from a fire hydrant on a hot day, winning a race, painting a picture, celebrating the harvest, watching a shiny-eyed child running up the driveway, childbirth itself. Remember joyful times in your life and remember how you *felt*—perhaps a quiet radiance or as if a light suddenly lit up within you so bright that you were barely able to contain it. Joy is the spontaneous recognition of our wholeness or holiness.

Joy may be an unexpected quality of the dying process you're both living. It can be there if you allow it, not making judgements that you shouldn't feel it.

Nurture your joy. Be a joyful servant. A very good 'goodbye' can be to live joy-fully.

Joy is the next step for humanity. A lot of people think we've been so unloving with each other and with the earth that the next step is more suffering. This is unnecessary if we see what happens in our lives, and in the world, as opportunities to learn instead of as punishment. Joy is the next step if we stop running away from pain. "Joy is your sorrow unmasked" (Kahlil Gibran). Resistance causes suffering. We don't have to resist the circumstances of our lives. And even if we *do*, eventually we'll get so fed up with the resulting suffering that we'll holler Uncle and just let go—*surrender*—which opens our hearts to joy. We may kick and struggle all the way home to joy—and we'll get there because it's the natural state of our being. We can't escape it.

If the person you're caring for is angry and looking for a target, you're likely to be one if you're radiating joy. "How can you be so happy when I'm here suffering?" We don't have to give up our joy for someone else. That's the old Guilt-Con Trick. You can explain that you're not happy they're suffering, but are happy to be with them and caring for them. Nourishing your joy is part of taking care of yourself so you can live *fully* through a dying process.

The joy I experienced caring for John, Mary, Dad, and other dying people was unexpected. It was the joy that comes from being open to someone else and seeing yourself in them. *A moment of spaciousness. A new awareness. An expansion of time. Nothing to do, nowhere to go, nobody to impress. Hearts opening. Two seemingly separate beings becoming one again.*

Guilt

I told you I was sick.

—epitaph on a tombstone

Guilt is a way we punish ourselves for not being perfect. It's a tool for manipulating ourselves and others.

Our culture's emphasis on both the past and the future promotes thinking like, *"If I'd just done something differently in the past, things would be better now."* And there we go screeching into guilt—the Monday morning quarterback rides again!

The underlying pattern of guilt is, "To be a good person, I should..." We are *intrinsically* good, valuable and worthy, and continue to be so, even if we *never* complete one 'should'. The established 'shoulds' may not be appropriate for our growth. If you complete a 'should' that is *not your own choice,* you are giving up your power and choosing to be a martyr or victim. A martyr is someone who thinks suffering is noble; a victim, someone who doesn't act on what their body, mind, feelings and soul tell them. Our choice is: not to complete a 'should' if it's not appropriate for us, or to change a 'should' to an "I want to . . ."

You become stronger each time you do what you *want* to do and *take responsibility for it.* Guilt, blame and punishment are ideas we need to let go of if we want to grow . . . or even to survive.

Because guilt makes us feel separate from each other and God, *self-forgiveness* is one of the most important things we can learn. We need to be as loving and compassionate with ourselves as we are with others—plus some, because people tend to be harder on themselves than on others. ("I forgive myself for anything I did that *now* seems unloving or unwise.") Each of us is what we can be in each moment of our lives, and we can be open to change. Once we forgive ourselves, no one can flog us with guilt.

A dying situation often brings up feelings of guilt, although caring for someone at home seems to help us avoid most of it. At home, there's time and a place to express whatever you now feel or have felt in the past . . . thereby avoiding later regrets and remorse from not having said or done what you might have. And if you have to take someone back to the hospital or nursing home, know you are worthy even if a home dying is more than you can handle. You can change "I *should* keep Grandma home" to "I'm a valuable person too, and I need assistance."

Besides not feeling guilty yourself, be careful not to make your patient feel guilty for dying. Saying, "I could go to the store if I didn't have to wait to give you your medicine," or "Don't leave me with all this," makes a person feel guilty and/or ashamed. Be aware of one pattern guilt takes: If we feel guilty about how we've treated someone, we sometimes make them look bad to justify our treatment of them!

Being honest with the dying person helps prevent guilt. (By this, I don't mean to go tell a dying husband or wife that you had an affair last year.) Honesty isn't ridding ourselves of guilt or getting ourselves off the hook at the expense of someone else.

One source of guilt is prevented by asking the patient what she or he wants whenever possible.

As I mentioned before, there's always the possibility that you'll do or give something to the person that will result in their death before you expect it. If you've earlier agreed to do your best, while knowing you can't know everything, you may prevent useless guilt. Remember my giving the "liver flush" to Mary? Spare yourself.

Be compassionate with yourself. *Forgive yourself...over and over again.* And instead of feeling guilt, congratulate yourself for outgrowing some old thought or feeling that is no longer appropriate for you, and for increasing in wisdom.

Humor

There are no tortuous roads to climb, for an instant of humor transports a soul into another world, a bright hopeful world where anything is possible. —a Deva

A friend found W.C. Fields on his deathbed reading the Bible and asked him why he was reading it. Fields answered, "I'm looking for loopholes."

Humor can cause a smile, a tiny chuckle or a big love-full belly laugh. Enjoy it. It's a source of deep nourishment for your voyage. Humor gives perspective to a world where it is seriously needed. If we can laugh together, we may be able to cry together and more. We can become one again. Whenever possible, try to see the humor in the situation you're facing now. As long as humor comes from your heart, it can't be harmful. Only cynicism and sarcasm have a destructive side.

Remember Charlie Chaplin? Remember how he increased our compassion for one another and reminded us of our common humanity? We laughed because he lightly showed us our conflicts and our pomposity. Laughing can be a great equalizer; it opens the heart.

Humor usually helps *unless* we use it to escape our feelings. A joke is a new vision, not just a way to mask pain or uncomfortableness.

Dying may be emotionally confusing for everyone involved. Humor helps us detach for a moment so we can see it more objectively. Humor helps the dying person deal with the frustration of needing help and not being able to do things she or he took for granted before. It helps him or her see their situation as less overwhelming and helps maintain a feeling of naturalness in the home. It releases blocked energies so we can see the larger picture. The details of life don't bog us down nearly so much if we laugh at ourselves, alone and together. We're really in a very leaky life-boat and we might as well enjoy it!

The belly laugh we had when Mary told us we were rushing her loosened the tension of many heavy days. The laugh we had when my sister told the priest that Dad was "somewhat" Catholic opened our hearts and lifted our fear. It would have been difficult to support them until they died without the lightening-up quality, the *levity,* of humor.

At a very deep level, humor heals.

Remember those funny old family stories together...Like the time Uncle Willie got caught... or Grandma found out....

Do you know why angels can fly? They take themselves lightly.

Anger

A bull in a small pen is likely to kick the fence down.
A bull in a large meadow has room to move.
　　　　　　　　　　　　　　　—Stephen Levine

Anger is an escape valve for the hurts and frustrations we pick up in the process of being human. We feel frustrated and hurt when we're attached to someone or something (life, for example) and things aren't going the way we think they should. ("I'm angry because I hurt because Dad *shouldn't* die.") Anger is a step on the way to surrender, a healthy sign as long as we don't hold on to it.

The amount of anger (or rage or violence) one feels is a measure of just how much hurt and frustration we're holding in. You can defuse anger by recognizing and expressing the hurt and frustration underneath it. Anger can be transformed into compassion by accepting that feeling angry is OK, by feeling and expressing the underlying hurt or frustration, and by accepting life as it *is* instead of holding on to how it *should be*. Again, we can't change something we don't first accept as real. For example, the anger I first felt when Dad was dying was transformed to compassion only after I'd thrown some plates and rocks and cried, and changed *"He shouldn't die"* to *"He is dying."*

It's perfectly natural to feel anger when you're supporting the dying process of someone you love. Your sense of loss, abandonment, insecurity, feeling that this dying is taking too long or that the person should feel grateful, etc., can bring up anger. You may feel anger when someone says they want to live and you feel they're not really trying. What they really may be saying is not "I want to live," but *"I'm afraid to die."* Sometimes with all this talk of acceptance and surrender, we feel angry if someone doesn't accept they're dying. Remember that *people can die with dignity and be angry down to the wire*. Perhaps that's a test for us. Do we really want them to die with dignity, their own way?

Let the anger out. The universe can absorb it. Our bodies can't. By not expressing anger we hang on to control, and the price is high. We can't see very clearly from inside hurt or anger. Unexpressed anger can turn into nagging, irritability, depression, high blood pressure and other serious illnesses or a big blow up later. Freeing it—accepting and expressing it—helps you and the dying person prepare for your loss and can help you both move toward acceptance. A dying person may not feel free to let go and die if people around are holding on to anger.

People often assume that expressing anger and hurting others are one and the same. It may be more hurtful *not* to express it. *Protecting* someone from anger says we don't trust them, that we know what's good for them. We're taking responsibility for *their* feelings and response, and assuming they're too dumb or unperceptive to recognize we're feeling anger. These things are a lot more hurtful than saying, "I'm angry with you. I love you and I'm angry."

If it's not appropriate for you to let out your anger in front of others, or you're afraid of the backlog of anger inside you, go off alone and bellow, throw balls, beat pillows, etc. If you have a wise friend or counselor, express the anger with them. Elisabeth Kübler-Ross suggests taking a foot and a half of rubber hose and beating on something you can't hurt until you can't beat anymore. I use the side of the bathtub. I prefer cleaning off black rubber marks to possibly cutting myself off from joy later.

It's all right for people, even children, to see us angry. Children need to know anger exists, what it's about, that it's OK to feel it, and how to deal with it. You can explain to children that you aren't angry at them or the person who's dying, but angry because you're frustrated and hurt. Let them know you can love someone and be angry at the same time. Encourage them to let out their anger in a way that doesn't physically hurt someone else. Maybe you could go off somewhere together and throw rocks. We lessen the amount of violence in the world by encouraging our children *and* everyone else to express their feelings.

I've heard people say about a dying person, "I'm angry because I love him so much." My response is, "Be angry. I know you love him and can continue to love him whether or not he's here in a body."

Hurt was probably the immediate cause of the anger; fear and loving conditionally the deeper causes (loving the person if she or he is here with me like I want).

We're moving toward loving unconditionally. "I love him including his need to die."

Fear

All know that the drops merge into the ocean
But few know that the ocean merges into the drops.
—Kabir

Dying and death may bring up more fear than any other circumstance of our lives. Supporting someone dying at home is an opportunity to face and accept this fear so we can transform it—and further open our hearts.

Fear makes us feel alone, like separate drops that are not part of an ocean. Fear is caused by judgements, mental commentaries on our experience that we project into the future, that prevent us from seeing the underlying unity of everything.

For example, if your experience was: *When I was seven my aunt died and I felt hurt and confused—Nobody would answer my questions and Mommy and Daddy acted strange.* The judgement probably was, *Dying is terrible* or *I'm afraid of death.* Even more likely, you didn't have a chance to experience that first mysterious death for yourself.

Parents' or friends' judgements—*Death is frightening* or *Dying is the worst thing that can happen*—were communicated verbally or non-verbally, leaving no possibility for you to experience dying and death *for yourself.* This is the way fear is passed from generation to generation. Your response to death from then on was probably controlled by a judgement you made at an early age.

And the judgements made in the past *rule* our lives until *we consciously* change them.

Descriptions, on the other hand, are not projected onto the future; they leave us free to experience the future as it comes. We can change a judgement—*I'm afraid of dying*—to a description, *Once my aunt died and I was afraid. I don't know how I'll feel the next time.* Or, *I know a lot of people are afraid of dying. I don't know how I feel because I haven't experienced it.* Changing a judgement to a description leaves our energies free for the freshness of each new moment.

Fear creates what it fears. We attract everything that lies in our energy field. We attract what we fear in order to give us an opportunity to look at, understand and release it. I was afraid of hospitals, blood, shots, sickness and death, so I was drawn to work with dying people in hospitals to transform those fears.

If you feel afraid of dying or of anything else, don't override the feeling by insisting, "I shouldn't feel it." Our feelings and instincts help us select the experiences that are right for us; if we ignore them we can end up with situations or people we don't like. Fear means we're not yet ready to accept an experience. Forcing an experience on yourself is not loving all of yourself unconditionally. As long as you force yourself to accept something you're not ready to accept, you'll feel separate and will find it difficult to accept other people and their feelings unconditionally.

When you feel afraid, feel the fear and don't assume that's all of who you are. It may help to say, "Oh, there's *that part of me* that's afraid of dying . . . of taking risks . . . of snakes" instead of "*I'm* afraid of dying . . . etc." Send love to the *part* of you that feels the fear and look for the judgement that caused it. Words like *good, bad, right, wrong, always, never, can't* and *should* often indicate a judgement. When you understand the judgement, you can release it by forgiving yourself for making it, and change it to a description. The next time you run into the same old fear, experiment with focusing on love instead of the fear. Over a period of time you'll find there are fewer things you're afraid of and you'll attract into your life fewer things you don't want.

We don't need fear. Fear is the absence of love. It can, however, show us where to shine love. "But," someone says, "fear warns me of danger!" Isn't it awareness or instinct for survival, not fear, that warns us of possible danger? "But I have to teach my children to fear knives and cars for their own safety." Teaching *with fear* is one way. Another is to use love and patience to help children understand that knives are neither good nor bad. They're useful to cut sandwiches and if used carelessly, they can cut us. We can help children understand potential dangers like knives and cars, and trust their survival instincts, or we can surround them with a miasma of our fear. Using love and patience we can help children understand dying without making it a fearful experience.

As you support a dying process, you may experience some of the fears of the dying person and some unique to being the one who remains behind in the everyday physical world. Fear is an initial response to losing control. Your fear about what life will be like without this person you love, particularly in a husband and wife relationship, is usually matched by his or her concern for you. How will you manage the children or the business? Talking together about fears and planning possible solutions and alternatives eases the adjustment to life without the other person. Talking together may also help a dying person accept death who feels afraid or guilty about deserting the family.

Your fear of loneliness matches their fear of loneliness. *"Here I am alone dealing with the daily problems of life"*/ *"Here I am alone, dying."* Share those feelings. *"I hurt because you're leaving me and going on"* / *"I hurt because I'm leaving you and going on."* Isolation, considered a major problem in the dying process, is greatly alleviated when your hearts are open to understanding each other's fears and pain. Facing your fear or resentment now—*"I'm not strong enough to stay here alone"* or *"I hate you for leaving me with this"*—prevents remorse later.

Worry comes from fear about what's happening now or what may happen in the future. Worry goes on inside our heads. If you feel worry coming up, take a few deep breaths, relax, breathe love *into your heart,* see if you're doing the best you know, and let go of the rest. This will give space for a new idea or solution to come to you. Or it just may be that whatever you're worrying about needs to happen to give someone an opportunity to learn from it.

Emotional Pain and Suffering

The amount of emotional pain and suffering around a dying is directly related to the fear around it. Fear makes us resist what's happening or may happen in our lives and the *resistance causes* emotional pain. When we stop resisting, stop seeing the world as we think it *should be,* emotional pain lifts. Suffering is a *habit* of pain, sadness or hurt. All of these are alleviated by accepting life as it *is.*

Pain is a useful message that tells us something in our lives is not working. It's no longer needed when we pay attention to it, locate the pattern or way of being that caused it and let go of it. When I was fighting against my dad's dying, I was in terrible pain. *Holding on* to him was obviously making me miserable. When I let go and accepted he was dying, I no longer hurt and was free to enjoy the time we had together.

Each journey to acceptance is unique; a lot of fear and arrogance made mine long and painful. Arrogance closes us to parts of life. Humility, being open, makes the journey a lot easier. While we're on our way, we need to be open to and accept our pain. Resisting pain just causes more pain; the pain is prolonged and becomes suffering. If we grieve right away when we hurt, we clean out most of the pain and don't suffer as much. If you're thinking, *"Well, I don't want to hurt but I do,"* accept what you feel. If you hurt you have to feel it before you can change it. After you've felt pain, you can begin to heal it by loving the *part* of you that feels it, releasing the *should* that caused it and not setting yourself up with more *shoulds.* (Some typical *shoulds* are: "He shouldn't die," "She should love me," "They should do things my way," "Life should be happier" and "Pain, starvation, pollution and war shouldn't exist.")

If we accept our pain, we can begin to accept someone else's pain. If we run away from our own, we'll run away from another's. Although we may be able to protect someone for awhile, in the long run it's impossible to protect anyone from emotional pain. We need it and create it until we accept life as it is. We often deny people the opportunity to learn surrender when we try to 'jolly' them out of their pain. Have you ever felt like hollering at someone who was denying your pain? "There's no reason to feel bad." "You shouldn't feel so sad." "I know exactly how you feel." "By next week... month... year you won't even remember." When someone says these things, people often respond with anger, which may distract them from feeling their pain and learning from it. Give the people you love a chance to feel their pain so they can learn from it and let go of it.

> Pain is the breaking of the shell that encloses your understanding. —Kahlil Gibran

Taking on someone else's pain is as useless as denying it. Then *two* people, not just one, are suffering and the world becomes darker. Every time a heart is glad it increases the light in the universe.

Taking on someone else's pain is one way to avoid feeling our own. (Something I did for most of my life.) Only when we clean out our own reservoir of pain can we support someone in pain without losing energy (burning out). What, then, can you do for someone who's hurting emotionally? Have compassion and share love. "I know you hurt and I love you." Once the person has felt the pain, if *they're* ready to release it, *possibly* you can help them see what they're resisting and suggest alternatives.

God doesn't pin a medal on us because we suffer. There may be part of ourselves that has an investment in our suffering ("If I suffer, I'm a good person." "If I suffer, I don't have to take responsibility for my life."). There may be a friend or relative who has an investment in your suffering ("If you were a good husband, you'd be suffering because your wife is dying."). **We express love by loving, not by suffering.**

Suffering is no longer a necessary part of the human experience. It has been useful to help us grow and we're moving toward growing by *awareness* instead of by pain. You can start looking for the pattern that could cause pain before you hurt or when you feel a little edgy. Waiting until we're in agony before we pay attention is a hard way to learn! It is possible to make a decision now, at this moment, in your *heart* to accept the circumstances of your life and you will never have to feel emotional pain again (unless, of course, you change the decision). As a friend of mine says of this possibility, "That's scarier than infinity!"

Before John and Mary died at home, I thought dying was mostly fear and suffering. There was much less of both than I'd projected. I found that being home with them and with Dad, and facing my fears and pain, opened my heart wider to my own love and wisdom. When I let go of the fear and pain I found them to be teachers about love and joy . . . and the path to opening the heart.

All distinctions are false: The moment you say, "This is good and that is bad," you have divided life and killed it.

—Lao-Tse

Chapter 9

Legal Considerations

The legal considerations around a pending death reflect the degree of complication in a person's life. They relate principally to how a person wants to distribute the property she or he has collected. The laws governing property distribution are complicated and vary from state to state. I can most usefully familiarize you with some of the terms and procedures you may meet.

Help the dying person get their business affairs in order. If you're not asked, ask if he or she needs help. It's often useful to have a *power of attorney,* a legal document that gives you authority to do things in someone else's name. This authority, which includes the right to sign the person's name, can be general or for a specific project only. Be sure to state in it, "I intend that this power of attorney last through a period of disability." In some states if you don't include this, a disability could invalidate it. You can buy a power of attorney form at a stationary store that sells pre-printed legal forms or write it yourself. Either way it must be signed in front of a notary public. Banks usually have a notary, or look in the Yellow Pages.

A *joint bank account* is also useful so you'll have cash available in case bank accounts or other assets are 'frozen' (can't be used) after death. Have available (if they exist) the person's will, insurance policies and key(s) to any safety deposit box(es).

Wills

A will is a legal document expressing how we want to distribute our material possessions and provide for our heirs upon our death. In legalese, a person who dies with a will dies *testate*.

Some of the advantages of making a will are: choosing the person we want to administer distribution of our property (called the executor, personal representative or personal rep), choosing who gets what (in case we doubt that survivors will follow our stated wishes), naming who will have custody of minor children, providing for an incapacitated adult, lessening the possibility of future legal disputes over property ownership. A will can also be a love letter to our heirs.

A person with small children and no spouse will probably die more peacefully having made clear arrangements for their care. Instead of blood relatives, many people name as guardian the person most likely to love and guide the child to adulthood in a way consistent with the parent's views.

If the *estate* (what we leave behind) is small, a will is not always necessary. Property jointly owned, joint or "pay on death" bank accounts, insurance proceeds, Series E Bonds, and death benefits like Social Security, VA and union benefits **bypass** a will.

If a person has a large estate, estate planning can save money in federal and state taxes. It's a complicated business which requires a lawyer who specializes in estate planning. Finding a 'good' lawyer may be difficult. Ask someone knowledgeable, such as a trust officer of a bank or an accountant, to recommend one or more lawyers they consider qualified in this area.

A simple will takes a lawyer from one to four hours to prepare by the time she or he talks with you, drafts the will and has it typed. Fees range from $50 to $75 *or more* per hour, so a simple will may cost between $75 and $300. *Before* meeting with a lawyer, ask how much he or she charges. If after the initial consultation you decide to retain the lawyer, reach a clear agreement on fees. If your income is low, check with a publicly supported legal clinic for no-cost or reduced fee services.

A VALID WILL

One of the main reasons to have a lawyer help write a will is to insure that it's valid (will stand up to a legal challenge). What constitutes a valid will differs from state to state. For many of us it seems simple. It's a piece of paper Grandpa writes saying to whom he wants to leave what. But the laws that determine the validity of a will place more importance on *form* than on content. A will *must* include property distribution, name a personal rep, and be signed and witnessed by two (sometimes three) people who sign in the presence of the author (testator) and each other.

A will may be partially or completely invalidated for many reasons: there were two witnesses instead of three; one of the witnesses forgot to write his address; the witness didn't attest that she knew it was a will she was witnessing; the husband or wife divorces and remarries, which revokes the part of the will related to the spouse; the author didn't sign all the pages; the author made handwritten changes on the will after it was formally executed, etc. Requirements such as these, set up to prevent fraud and to insure that a property owner's wishes are carried out, probably catch only a minimal number of crooks. And lawyers who make money because of the laws about wills are not likely to initiate legislation to change the laws that exist.

So, we have enormous latitude in the *provisions* of our wills, but not in the *form*. Check the specific requirements in your state.

HOLOGRAPHIC WILLS

A holographic will is one that is signed, dated and written *entirely by hand by the author*. It must include disposal of property and name a personal rep. No witness is required. It's recognized as valid in the following states: Alaska, Arizona, Arkansas, California, Idaho, Kentucky, Louisiana, Mississippi, Montana, Nevada, North Carolina, North Dakota, Oklahoma, Pennsylvania, South Dakota, Tennessee, Texas, Utah, Virginia, West Virginia, Wyoming, Maryland (if written by someone serving in the armed services) and New York (if written by a soldier, sailor or mariner).

So, if you live in one of these states and don't own property in another you can write your own will. A person who has property in more than one state needs a lawyer. In some of the states listed, it may be possible to type or dictate a holographic will. Check with the court in your area that has probate jurisdiction.

NO WILL

A lot of people die *intestate,* which means without a will. When people die without a will, their property is distributed according to the *law of intestate succession* of the state in which they live. Property jointly owned, life insurance proceeds and death benefits *bypass* the law of intestate succession.

Under laws of intestate succession, property generally goes first to the surviving husband or wife, then to their children and then to other blood relatives. If you care who gets your possessions, it's a good idea to find out the law in your state so you don't create problems for your survivors. A legal clinic or lawyer can help you.

In some states, for example, if you have a wife and one minor child, the law distributes half of the estate to your wife and half to the child. If the child is a minor, the court will name a guardian, who is normally the surviving parent. *But the* guardian may have to put up a bond (post money) and *must* get permission from the court to spend any of the child's money, and must file an accounting with the court each year. This means time, money and nuisance for the guardian, which can be avoided by writing a will.

For the enjoyment of it and/or to avoid dealing with lawyers and courts, some people simply give away their property before they die. Legally we must file a federal gift tax return on all gifts given to one person worth over $10,000 per year (or $20,000 per year if the spouse agrees). Each year we can give tax-free as many gifts of this size to as many people as we choose. If one gives larger gifts and dies before filing the tax return, the personal rep is responsible for filing it.

The Personal Representative

Personal Representative is the new name for *executor,* the person named by the writer of the will to take charge of his or her financial affairs and distribute property after death. If there is no will, the personal rep is named by the court. The work of a personal rep may take several years if the estate is large or complicated. She or he is paid by the will writer's estate for the work done. The payment varies by state; it is 'a reasonable fee' or a percentage (1% to 5%) of the estate.

The following discussion of the legal responsibilities of the personal rep is excerpted from *Law for the Layman* by attorney George G. Coughlin:

1. *He (she) may take the assets of the estate into his (her) possession.* (This means the personal rep takes control of the assets of the estate and obtains full information about all the deceased's belongings. She or he opens a bank account in the name of the estate and transfers the deceased's accounts to his or her name as personal rep. She or he collects the proceeds from insurance policies and looks after stocks and bonds. Reps need to keep detailed records of all financial proceedings.)

2. *He (she) may sell and liquidate personal property and convert the assets of the estate into cash.* (If cash is needed to pay debts, the personal rep can sell personal property and real estate.)

3. *He (she) may pay debts and funeral and administration expenses.* (This involves placing a notice in newspapers that any creditors of the deceased present their claims. If state and federal taxes are due, the rep is responsible for paying them.)

4. *He (she) may distribute the estate to the beneficiaries.*

Probate

Probate is the name used for the personal rep's work and for the procedure of opening and closing an estate. It documents legal ownership of inherited property. According to Phillip Stern, author of *Lawyers on Trial,* "Probate is up to 100 times more expensive here than in England, and that's because England 'delawyered' the process. In this country we end up paying two and a half to three times as much in fees to probate attorneys as we do in funeral expenses."

Probate is necessary if a person dies with a will, or with property such as real estate, stocks and bonds, bank accounts, etc., that must be passed on according to the laws of interstate succession. It's *not* necessary if a person leaves no will and only owns property of the sort that bypasses the law of *intestate* succession (like jointly owned property, joint or "pay on death" bank accounts, insurance proceeds, Series E Bonds and death benefits like Social Security, VA and union benefits). Legally, personal effects and clothing may be subject to probate, but in practice they're generally divided among friends and relatives.

If your relative or friend dies and you know she or he has a will, take it out of the shoe box, safety deposit box or wherever it's been kept. You or your lawyer should then take it and a copy of the death certificate to your local court with probate jurisdiction and file for probate. The judge will decide if the will is valid. If your relative or friend dies without a will and there is property that doesn't bypass the law of intestate succession, you or your lawyer should take the death certificate to the court and file to be name personal rep. The judge decides if you're the proper person for the job. If appointed, you may be required to post a bond to guarantee that you'll do a good job and won't run off with the loot.

Once you file, the court issues *letters testamentary* if there is a will or *letters of administration* if there is not. The 'letters' state that the personal rep accepts responsibility for collecting assets, paying debts and taxes, distributing the property and closing the estate.

The personal rep *lists* the assets collected, the debts, inheritance taxes and the share of each beneficiary. If there are no disputes, the property is distributed to the beneficiaries; they acknowledge receiving their share and the estate is closed. If there are disputes, the estate can be settled by written agreement among the disputing parties, or the personal rep and the people involved go before the judge for a decision. Upon proof of distribution, the estate can be closed.

Taxes

Depending on the size of the estate, state and/or federal taxes may have to be paid. Taxes vary from state to state. A few impose none.

As of 1984, a federal tax return must be filed on any *gross estate* that exceeds $325,000. The limit will be raised to $400,000 in 1985, $500,000 in 1986, and $600,000 in 1987 and thereafter. *Gross estate* means everything someone owned, or got rid of but kept some control over, and includes all things, such as joint property, that bypass probate. The tax return must be filed and is due within nine months of the death, although you can apply for an extension.

Federal estate tax laws are complicated to begin with, and they have recently undergone major revisions, so check with the IRS. If there is an estate of any size, you should consult an attorney or accountant. You should be aware (since some lawyers are not) that the IRS no longer requires filing a preliminary estimate of assets.

What estate planning is really about, besides seeing that a person's property is well managed and properly distributed, is *saving money on taxes.* Tax accountants, bank trust officers and estate planning lawyers are the people to consult if the finances involved warrant it. They know, for example, how to use trusts, marital deductions and similar devices to 'split' an estate so that upon the death of the husband or wife federal estate taxes will be at a lower rate. Many of us who aren't knowledgeable about taxes think owning everything in common when we're married is the loving way to handle property. However, for people with a large estate, joint ownership may be unwise because it increases the estate taxes that may be due in the future.

Two publications available at your local IRS office may be helpful: #559, *Tax Information for Survivors, Executors and Administrators,* and #448, *A Guide to Federal Estate and Gift Taxation.*

Living Wills

People are beginning to realize that each of us has the right to determine the nature of our own death. A number of states, including New Mexico, Texas, California, Nevada, Oregon, Idaho, Arkansas, Kansas, Washington and North Carolina, have passed what are generally called "Right to Die" laws. These laws establish clear legal guidelines to protect our right to refuse medical procedures which serve only to prolong the dying process. They also protect doctors from liability for acting in accordance with our wishes. (For a comparison of these state laws, see Appendix E.)

These laws allow anyone to sign a document stating that if she or he is suffering from a terminal illness that is certified by one (or two) doctors, his or her life should not be sustained by medication, artificial means or heroic measures. Such a document is often called a *Living Will.*

It's encouraging that many people are reclaiming an age-old right that had been given away to doctors, lawyers and courts. None of them has the right to say how long a patient or their family must suffer, or that a family potentially must go broke. A Living Will relieves both family and doctors of responsibility for making the ultimate decision about some-body else's life. In a home dying sustaining life artificially usually is not a problem. It might become one if a person had to go into a hospital for renal dialysis or other specific treat-ment and while there their condition worsened or they went into a coma. So, even if a person plans to die at home, making a Living Will can be useful.

I suggest making a Living Will even if you live in a state that has not yet passed a Right to Die law. In the event of a legal, ethical or medical question about a treatment, it would serve as clear evidence of your wishes. Doctors may feel safer about being sued for malpractice if there's a Living Will. Although there has not yet been a court decision affirming that these wills are legally enforceable (outside of states that have passed legislation), there are a growing number of cases which affirm that patients have the *right to refuse treatment,* whether or not this results in death.

If you are a Catholic, you may already be aware that a June 1980 Declaration of Euthanasia concluded: "When inevitable death is imminent, it is permitted in conscience to take the decision to refuse forms of treatment that would only secure a precarious and a burdensome prolongation of life." Protestant groups have made similar statements.

Concern for Dying, a nonprofit organization, researched the subject of what effect a Living Will might have on a life insurance policy. They reported that signing a Living Will would not invalidate any life insurance policy and would not be construed as an intent to commit suicide. Insurance com-panies stand to save a lot of money if people are not kept alive artificially for months or years in a hospital.

To My Family, My Physician, My Lawyer and All Others Whom It May Concern

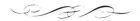

Death is as much a reality as birth, growth, maturity and old age—it is the one certainty of life. If the time comes when I can no longer take part in decisions for my own future, let this statement stand as an expression of my wishes and directions, while I am still of sound mind.

If at such a time the situation should arise in which there is no reasonable expectation of my recovery from extreme physical or mental disability, I direct that I be allowed to die and not be kept alive by medications, artificial means or "heroic measures". I do, however, ask that medication be mercifully administered to me to alleviate suffering even though this may shorten my remaining life.

This statement is made after careful consideration and is in accordance with my strong convictions and beliefs. I want the wishes and directions here expressed carried out to the extent permitted by law. Insofar as they are not legally enforceable, I hope that those to whom this Will is addressed will regard themselves as morally bound by these provisions.

Signed_____

Date _____

Witness_____

Witness_____

Copies of this request have been given to _____

_____

_____

_____

Living Will prepared by Concern for Dying

If you live in a state that has passed a Right to Die law, write to the Society for the Right to Die, 250 West 57th Street, New York, NY, for the form preferred by your state. Try to enclose a donation of $2 or more.

If your state has not yet passed a version of this law, you may send for a copy of a Living Will, like the sample shown here, by mailing a donation of $2 or more to Concern for Dying at the *same address* as the Society for the Right to Die. If you ask, they will also send a mini-will (condensed version of the Living Will) to keep in your wallet in case of an accident.

You can alter the wording of a Living Will form to suit your needs and desires, but it's a good idea to check with a knowledgeable attorney. The will should be witnessed by at least two people and notarized to show the seriousness with which you regard the statement. It wouldn't hurt to update it every few years by redating it and initialing the new date.

Once you sign a Living Will, to be sure it's enforced, *let everyone close to you know how you feel.* Talk with your doctor or clergyman and give him or her a copy. Tell your family and be sure they know where you've put it. If you doubt that your family or doctor will follow your wishes, talk with a lawyer.

Body Donations

In recent years all states have enacted or revised Anatomical Gift Laws, which permit people to donate all or parts of their bodies to a hospital, research or educational institution. If you or the dying person want to give your body or parts of it, state this in the will or fill out a Uniform Donor Card or other such document. Call a medical school or hospital to get the exact details for your state and area. Ask if your age and physical condition is suitable. Be sure family members' wishes are known, as well as the document's location.

Uniform Donor Cards are available from some medical schools. A number of states include them on the backs of driver's licenses. (See Appendix A for other sources.)

UNIFORM DONOR CARD

OF _____

Print or type name of donor

In the hope that I may help others, I hereby make this anatomical gift, if medically acceptable, to take effect upon my death. The words and marks below indicate my desires.

I give: (a)_____any needed organs or parts

(b)_____only the following organs or parts

_____

Specify the organs or parts

for the purposes of transplantation, therapy, medical research or education;

(c)_____my body for anatomical study if needed.

Limitations or special wishes, if any: _____

Signed by the donor and the following two witnesses in the presence of each other:

_____   _____
Signature of Donor   Date of Birth of Donor

_____   _____
Date Signed   City & State

_____   _____
Witness   Witness

This is a legal document under the Uniform Anatomical Gift Act or similar laws.

For further information consult your local memorial society or:

Continental Association of Funeral & Memorial Societies
1828 L Street, N.W. Washington, D.C. 20036

Separate nothing out as less sacred than anything else.
Everything and everyone is equally divine.
                        —*from a meditation on the Christ*

Chapter 10

Healing

At the core of healing lies a deep mystery that is to be respected. It is the mystery of transformation and regeneration and is different for each person. It is the mystery of balance and harmony, and at the core of this mystery lies the universal Heart.

—Satya Miriam
Healing is Transformation

I share with you my beliefs about the nature of our being, of disease and of healing. Throughout the world increasing numbers of people are coming to the same or similar realizations. They are departures from a lot of old assumptions.

Each of us is a whole composed of body, mind, feelings and soul. Body, mind and feelings are sometimes called the 'body', or personality of the soul. The word 'personality' comes from the Latin *persona,* which means 'mask'. Soul is spirit, or God individualized.

Disease (dis-ease) indicates a disharmony within the whole. The body is the last part of us in which dis-ease manifests. It appears first as a disharmony between the soul and mind or feelings. To heal, we have to understand and treat ourselves as whole beings within a physical and social environment.

At present, most medical doctors are trained to treat the symptoms of disease rather than to support an individual's own process of healing. Penicillin and aspirin, for example, are not going to heal a person's real dis-ease. At best they buy time by curing symptoms so one can discover and heal the real imbalance. Splints may help cure a leg broken in a car accident, but they won't heal the consciousness that *caused* the person to be in the accident. Curing symptoms and healing dis-ease aren't the same thing.

The more we have given away the *responsibility* for our health to doctors, the sicker we've become. It's not the doctors' fault. We're the ones who got addicted to the body as our main point of reference and mistakenly looked for the source of healing outside of ourselves. *The source of healing is within.* The work of medical doctors can be valuable, but has limits because it works only on the body. The exception is psychiatrists who generally work with mental and emotional symptoms. *Real healing must take place at all levels of our being.*

Healing, *righting* the energy balance within us, is a process that requires our active participation. Human beings are dense, somewhat solidified energy. An imbalance in this energy results in disharmony or disease. It can be a great adventure to find the source of the imbalance and to heal ourselves. The person you are supporting in the dying process can certainly be healed—even if his or her body cannot be cured. Sometimes an imbalance is healed and the body dies anyway.

Many people have lost faith in prayers (an aid to healing) when they prayed for someone to be healed and she or he died. Their prayer *was* heard. Perhaps they didn't recognize it was answered. The disharmony may have been healed and it was time to leave an uninhabitable body. Prayer is useful if we avoid praying for what we *want* and pray instead for whatever is the *highest good* for ourselves or others.

We're fortunate if we know the Divine Plan for ourselves, let alone for someone else.

We are either victims of our diseases or we are responsible for them. I believe we're responsible. This is much more hopeful and useful than thinking we're victims. If we're victims, disease is out of our control and we can't do anything about it except try to cure the symptoms. On the other hand, if we are responsible (accept our dis-ease as ours), it is possible to heal ourselves.

The principal pitfall when we begin to take responsibility for our dis-ease is guilt. Who needs to feel sick *and* guilty too? For many years parts of me were sick. For four of those years, after I was introduced to holistic healing and began to take responsibility for my sickness, I felt like a spiritual leper. I didn't want to see anyone because I was sure they would see I was sick and know something was wrong with me spiritually. I felt sick and I felt guilty—and I was afraid to talk with anyone about it.

Spare yourself! There's nothing to feel guilty about. The body is a sacred vehicle and messenger. If the postman brought you a letter that contained information you didn't want to hear, you wouldn't berate the postman or feel guilty. When our bodies give us a message that something is not working, instead of berating ourselves, we can thank our bodies, send them love, take care of them in the way appropriate for us and start looking for the source of the imbalance.

Within each of us is soul and body (which includes mind and feelings), man and woman, giver and receiver, pragmatist and visionary, do-er and be-er, father and mother, creator and inspiration, light and darkness, intellect and intuition, movement and rest, will and awareness. When we balance these polarities, we feel vibrant, alive and whole. If we neglect any of them, we cause an imbalance in the whole—dis-ease. We can balance them by accepting, nourishing and expressing them. The marriage of the polarities within us is the most important marriage we make. It opens our hearts and more.

To find the *source* of the imbalance, we must find the part or parts of ourselves that we're not loving unconditionally. When body, mind and feelings are not in balance, we limit the amount of God (energy) we can express, and we are not aware of who we really are. If we accept only *body*, we accept only half of ourselves, of God. If we accept only *soul*, we accept only half. When we accept both we are truly healthy, conscious of our *God-self*.

You may want to look at the polarities in your own being. Are you listening to both your visionary and your pragmatist? Are you using your intellect as well as your intuition? If you're a woman, are you allowing the man in you to express itself? If you're a man, are you expressing the woman in you? Are you allowing time for quiet and time for activity, time for creating and time for inspiration? Are you as good at receiving as you are at giving and vice-versa? Are you loving and accepting all of yourself?

> *When you make the two one, and when you make the inner as the outer, and the outer as the inner, and the above as the below, and when you make the male and the female into a single one, so that the male will not be male and the female not be female, then shall you enter the Kingdom.*
>
> —Jesus Christ in
> *The Gospel According to Thomas*

We can recognize *imbalances* where we see sickness instead of health, fear instead of love, hate instead of compassion, separation instead of unity, war instead of peace. Imbalance exists when we don't see matter and spirit as equally sacred, and when we don't accept life as it is. Balance comes from changing what we can and leaving the rest to be transformed in its own time. An imbalance exists if we don't remember, *"Not my will but Thine."*

What can you do if you find you have a life-threatening disease? An anonymous contributor to an article in *New Age Magazine* gives some useful advice. The first point is particularly directed to people who have cancer.

1. Run, don't walk, away from 95% of medical paraphernalia and practice. *(For some physical problems this is not true. A team of medical and holistic doctors would be most useful.)*

2. Sit down and center yourself. Begin reversing the self-irresponsibility pattern endorsed by the culture and ask yourself, 'How did I create this situation? Do I really want out? Of life, of the disease?' If you decide it's life you want out of, acknowledge that cancer was the one-way ticket you purchased . . . If you decide you want out of the disease, then accept that any condition you have created can be recreated. Any decision you have made can be reversed.

3. Take a holistic approach . . . A superior healer, to use the Chinese phrase, uses modalities that support the healing forces of the patient; the inferior healer uses modalities that fight disease. Locate a superior healer.

4. Use your experience as a learning and growth vehicle by extracting the principles involved . . . it is not enough to live. Survival as a life purpose is mockery. The body, like a fine musical instrument that must be kept in tune in order to serve as a constructive influence, might occasionally need repairing and tuning. When it no longer responds to repairing and tuning, it should be discarded as graciously and as soon as possible. Clutter diminishes the clarity of living.

You may want to consider healing possibilities you haven't tried before or you may want to stay with the familiar. The following list gives some of the tools you can use to create your unique path of integration. After learning something about the various tools, find the ones appropriate for you by using your intuition and choosing from the heart. (See Appendix F.)

Allopathy	Homeopathy	NeoReichean work
Yoga	Do-in	Dancing
Herbs	Shiatsu	Drawing

Rolfing	Polarity therapy	Dreams
Feldenkrais	Psychic surgery	Rebirthing
Vitamins	Chiropractic	Bach flowers
Diet	Aikido	Meditation
Jogging	Biofeedback	Affirmations
Acupuncture	Gestalt therapy	Astrology
Massage	Encounter	Tarot
Color work	Psychosynthesis	Guided meditation
Sound	Aura balancing	Prayer
Music	Tai Chi	Spiritual healers

I've often seen people begin to experiment with alternative techniques and become discouraged when they didn't see the desired results. Either the person didn't work on *all* levels (body, mind, feelings and soul) or didn't know that a person can be healed but no longer need a body. Healing as an intellectual pursuit alone doesn't work.

There are a number of survey books on natural and holistic healing: *The Holistic Health Handbook,* by the Berkeley Holistic Health Center; *The Practical Encyclopedia of Natural Healing,* by Mark Bricklin; *Holistic Medicine: Introduction and Overview,* by James S. Gordon, M.D. (published by the U.S. Government and available through the Institute of Noetic Sciences, 600 Stockton Street, San Francisco, CA 94108).

Calling in the Light

In my experience, one technique of healing which works is to *call in the Light.* Light is the energy that created and sustains us. It is another name for unconditional love. When we call in the Light (become conscious of it), we *become* the Light for as long as we remain focused in our hearts. The purpose of calling it in is to support healing.

If you want to support yourself or another with the Light, ask that it be present. I ask that "the Spirit of the Living Love and Light be present." Use words that suit you. There's no need to tell the Light what to do because it has perfect knowledge. Ask that it be used for the 'highest good' of whomever you're sending it to so you don't interfere with their process or your own. You may feel it or see it as a light coming through the top of your head and filling your body. No effort is needed. When we exert ourselves, we have no place to receive. At first you may feel a little dizzy and uneasy. This passes as your body adjusts to the energy.

Holding the Light means remaining focused in your heart for whatever amount of time feels good. This may be a few minutes or a half hour. At the same time as you hold the Light for another, you are also being healed. I find holding the Light very supportive for dying people and continue to do it periodically during the first weeks after death.

Laws for Healing

Three universal laws for healing are: 'As above, so below', self-forgiveness, and 'As a man thinketh in his heart, so he is'.

As above, so below. If there is perfection at the level where we are One, we individuals are capable of it as well. We can transform each cell of our body to radiant health by calling the Light into each cell, by visualizing each cell as perfect and by forgiving ourselves for having thought it could be otherwise. If there is total love, beauty, peace and joy 'above', they're here as well. We have to lift the blinders that prevent us from seeing them. Simple, and yet not easy.

The blinders are our *judgements.* "This is good (or bad)." "This is right (or wrong)." *Everything is energy and energy is neither right nor wrong.* It just is. All energy is One, God. And it can be used skillfully or unskillfully. Judgements make things seem separate so people feel there's more than One. A table, flower or bomb are all manifestations of the one energy. We have free will to use energy as we choose.

Self-forgiveness. God has nothing to forgive us for because we were never judged in the first place. However, *we* make judgements so we need to forgive *ourselves.* We can forgive ourselves as many times a day as we need to. Each time we do we open our hearts. *"I forgive myself for being afraid I don't know enough to write this book; I forgive myself for thinking there isn't enough money for my needs; I forgive myself for not being more loving with myself and others."*

Self forgiveness is an art people learn as they move toward loving themselves and remembering who they are. (A useful pamphlet called *Self-Forgiveness: An Act of Life,* by Robert Waterman, is available from the Southwestern College of Life Sciences. See Appendix A for the address.)

As a man thinketh in his heart, so he is. This goes for women too! Energy follows thought. We create what we think. If we think we're sick, we're sick. And we have free will to change our thinking. If we think from *our hearts,* we're healthy. If we think from our hearts, we know love, joy, peace, beauty and abundance. Even if we just focus on these qualities with our minds we make space for them to develop in our lives. We can choose each day what and from where we will think. Will we create love and beauty around us or create fear, sadness, scarcity and loneliness? When I find myself thinking in negative circles in my head, I say "God" to short-circuit it. This might work for you too. Try it.

If your body is sick, you might ask all your friends to think of and visualize you as healthy, not sick. A lot of friends thinking of you as sick can hold you to old patterns and help you stay sick.

If a person has cancer, she or he can visualize each cell working perfectly and any malfunctioning cells lifting up and out of the body. Again, *remember* to work at the feeling, body and soul levels as well. Carl Simonton, M.D., and his wife Stephanie, a therapist, of Ft. Worth, Texas, have worked extensively and successfully with meditative and visualization techniques for cancer and have instruction tapes available. See Appendix A for their address.

A Guided Meditation

Guided meditation is another way to explore our inner experience and capacity for healing. Earlier I mentioned that a transcendent or mystical experience can eliminate or transform pain. Guided meditation is a simple method of helping someone get in touch with their own transformative energies, whether or not they're in pain. Use the meditation below or create one that's right for the particular circumstances of the person you're guiding. You may give or receive a guided meditation. Don't be upset if the person cries. People often do. Some people fall asleep and that's OK too. Both times I used this meditation with Mom and Dad they fell asleep about the time they got to the 'top of the mountain'... and they woke up feeling great!

Ask the person to lie down or sit, making him or herself as comfortable as possible. Keep your voice soft and non-interfering. Leave time (long pauses) as you read for the person to get images and experience his or her feelings. The meditation:

Close your eyes and breathe gently. With each breath gently move deeper inside yourself... Imagine that you're in a beautiful meadow... The sun is coming down in golden rays through you and around you. (If the person is in pain, suggest: *As you feel the sun, allow its light to move through any place in your body that hurts... any place in your feelings that hurt... start relaxing the tension around the hurt ... Imagine each cell around that area softening... opening ... relaxing... Keep softening and opening and letting the light fill you... Then continue.*)

Open fully to the light and let it fill you... Relax and feel the richness around you and through you... Smell the air ... Touch the earth and feel it in your hands... are there birds... or flowers... or animals...? Be with them... You feel perfectly comfortable with everything... Is there a stream or brook?... If so, listen to the sound of the water. Are there any wild berries... wild strawberries or anything to eat?... If so, put it in your mouth and really savor it... If there is anything you want to do in this meadow, where there are no limits, do it... explore... sing... dance...

On the other side of the meadow is a beautiful mountain ... start walking toward it and climbing up it... If you need help, imagine something to help you... a bird, a person, an elevator. You can imagine anything you want... You can see that the light at the top of the mountain is incredibly beautiful... As you climb, the light starts to fill you. Soon you're at the top. If you need a rest, invent a seat... An exquisite beam of light surrounds you and fills you... allow yourself to really feel the light... Within the light, a figure or form comes toward you that represents the highest you know... You feel this being's love for you... really let that love in... (allow plenty of time)... You know that this person or energy has always loved you and has never judged you or anything you've done... Forgive yourself for all the times you've judged yourself or other people... for all the times you've felt unworthy... guilty... fearful.

As you forgive yourself, feel your heart opening wider ... Forgive yourself for all the judgements you made against your body... your feelings... your mind... Allow forgiveness and love to fill every cell of your being... If you like, ask the figure or energy any question you have about anything ... The figure or energy reaches out to you and gives you a gift to take with you so you can remember this experience... After you receive the gift, say goodbye, knowing you can always return... From the top of the mountain take the light that fills you and radiate it to everyone... all the people you love... all the people, plants, animals... all the creatures of the earth... When you feel ready, slowly come down the mountain with your heart open, bringing this light energy with you... Take all the time you need; there's no hurry... When you feel ready, open your eyes, bringing the energy back into this room.

Allow yourself to receive and share whatever the person brings back.

Butterflies count not in months but in moments and have time enough.

—Rabindranath Tagore

Chapter 11

Preparation for Death and Afterward

For brief as water falling will be death.
—Conrad Aiken

Signs of Imminent Death

As the moment of death approaches, a dying person usually wants more and more time alone, resting and sleeping, preparing internally for what is to come. Cells are dying at a greater rate than ever and the person has less and less physical energy. As you see the person less connected to the outer world, it's useful if there are fewer visitors and distractions.

You may find it nourishing at times to just sit quietly and watch the dying person. Silence is a living, healing energy that makes space for renewal and internal preparations. One friend said, "I know why I was sitting with my father. It was so my heart could open wider and I could see his essence." Your intuition will tell you if gentle touching is a comfort to the person or an intrusion.

Don't misinterpret a dying person's seeming distance or lack of connectedness with you as a lack of love. Even as they love you dearly, they begin to move on toward the new life.

Share this with family members whose feelings might be hurt. While death is easy, dying can be hard work.

Dying people are often conscious until death. Some move into a coma. Although medically they're called unconscious, they're not. As I said before, a person in this state hears everything at some level. Talk in their presence as you would with a conscious person, not as if they were unconscious. We are alive and have consciousness even when very little or nothing is functioning outwardly.

If you have unfinished things to share with someone in a coma, talk to them and know they will hear you. Questions are generally fruitless because the person can't answer verbally. Although, if you listen with your heart, you may hear the answer. One way to see a coma is as a kindly teaching that we are not just a body.

The dying person will take less and less food and liquid. Less urine will be eliminated. If she or he can no longer eat or drink, keep their mouth as moist and fresh as possible. As I mentioned before, ice chips or a wet washcloth to suck on are useful. Lemon glycerine swabs may be satisfying or may taste too strong.

If a person is dehydrated or if the air is very dry, mist his or her room with a plastic spray bottle filled with water—an emptied Windex bottle will do. Some people enjoy having their bodies sprayed with a water mist. Ask.

One sign of approaching death, but not necessarily imminent death, may be an odor coming from the person. To me, it seems to be the smell of cells decaying. If there are lung complications, the odor *may* be particularly strong. With cancer, a strong odor is sometimes present earlier. In John's case the odor was so strong that some of us felt nauseous. Burning incense and putting Tiger Balm under our noses helped. Ben-Gay works as well. In my father's case, by contrast, there was no odor.

A person in the last stages of dying may find massage soothing or an intrusion or interruption. Use your intuition. A very gentle massage may be one of the last outward ways of expressing your love. Dying people are sensitive to pressure. A person with cancer may be quite 'skeletal' by now with very little fleshy protection for the bones. (Remember pillows and padding between the knees.) Because the skin is also sensitive, use a cream skin toughener if you have one. I've used Lanacane and an oil prepared by an herbologist containing Benzoin and myrrh. Sensitivity to light may be heightened. If you need a bright light to see by, warn the person so they're prepared for it.

As people approach death, their arms and legs may get colder and colder as circulation withdraws. Keep them warmly covered. Some people sweat profusely. If they do, lighten the covers. Don't tuck in the top sheet or covers so the person can move about if she or he is able. Again, you may be asked to turn the person frequently, which can be exhausting and may take two people. Most people close to death need less pain medication.

Other signs that death is probably near: the underside of the body becoming a darker color, the mouth hanging open, brown secretions in the mouth (old blood possibly from the stomach lining), the pupils of the eyes reacting less to changes in light. The person may have a glazed faraway look or stare into the distance without blinking. In sleep the eyes may shut only partially. If you take a pulse (a measure of the heartbeat) you may notice it's weak. The skin may be pale and waxy and the face drawn. Again, even if the person is showing very few signs of life, talk in their presence as if they're present, because they are.

As a result of changes in body metabolism, the dying person may experience increasing confusion about time, place and the identity of family and friends. Reassure them by telling them the time, a person's name or who's in the room. Loosening connections here is part of a person's preparation for death. It's important not to insist that she or he pay attention to what's 'real' for us and which may no longer be for them.

It's not uncommon for dying people to talk out loud with God or someone who has already died. Dad saw lights around him. Some people may call this hallucinating; I prefer not to use the word because it suggests they're crazy or need sedation. They aren't and they don't. I believe they've just opened the door to another reality. The person may be having a profound religious or mystical experience. Stanislav Grof and Joan Halifax, *The Human Encounter with Death,* report, "Dying individuals quite regularly experience various degrees of age regression and relive important memories or review their entire lives." Respect these preparations.

As a person moves close to death, his or her breathing usually becomes more and more labored. Secretions may build up in the lungs so that less oxygen is being exchanged for carbon dioxide, further weakening the person physically. You can help them by speaking gently and soothingly, or just by breathing gently and fully yourself. You might ask the person to remember how they breathed sitting or sleeping next to someone they love and suggest they try to breathe that way now. Even closer to death the breathing pattern may change again. A drastic change in breathing doesn't mean the person is going to die immediately. A person may continue for a number of days to breathe in a way that might lead you to guess that each breath is the last. The breathing may seem pretty bizarre and frightening if you're not used to hearing it. There may be a crescendo of breath and then no breathing for 10-30 seconds. Doctors call this Cheyne-Stokes or neurogenic breathing. You may hear a rasping or gurgling sound at the back of the throat caused by oral secretions that the person can't cough up. *Elevating the person's head may help ease the effort of breathing.*

If the breathing bothers you, take breaks out of the room. The breathing may not only sound strange, but can bother us because we feel helpless. Perhaps the deeper reason for our discomfort is that by now we're seeing the difference between a person and his or her body. When we see the body hanging on, we feel a sense of inappropriateness. Remember, you're really just watching the labor pains of the soul.

The symptoms of imminent death given here may not all appear at the same time and some may never appear.

Dying people know at some level when they're going to die. Both Mary and Dad communicated that they knew. Using your intuition is one way to know when death will come. When John was dying, I meditated and prayed for guidance and was told he had four days. On the fourth day he died. Don't worry if you're 'off'. God's timetable is flexible.

Whether or not a person has accepted that they're dying, there is frequently a period of peace before death—perhaps it's that final surrender. It is interesting to note that according to V. Ruth Gray, a nurse and author of *Dealing with Death and Dying,* "a dying person always turns his head toward the light." Could it be that as we die we know we're going home to the Light even before we open the garden gate?

Being with Someone the Last Few Days

The last few days your attitude needs to be one of letting go and releasing the person. Both of you are working on surrender, trusting the moment. Suffering is caused if a person is ready to die and he or she feels the family is hanging on. It creates a struggle. *"I know I can't stay and I don't feel like I can leave."* Let the person know you'll be OK and encourage him or her to go free.

At this point all we can be is present. Quiet. Loving. Open. Holding hands if that feels right. We can hold the Light (page 213). Suggest she or he breathe as calmly as possible. I suggest (verbally or non-verbally) that the person move toward the Light, allowing him or herself to feel lighter and lighter, lifting up. See if the meditation that follows is useful for you.

Two situations that may come up at the end of a dying process can generate a lot of guilt if we misunderstand them. The first is a feeling of irritation or anger that this process is taking so long. It's a natural feeling a lot of us experience, like that of a mother who loves her child yet is tired because she or he needs so much attention. Recognize the anger or irritation and forgive yourself. (See Anger, page 184.) These feelings are signals that we need rest, a change of scene, time away for ourselves. The person is still here because he or she needs to finish something on some level. It'll be easier for you if you don't make assumptions about how long the process will take and continue to pace yourself.

The second situation occurs if the death happens while you're out of the house or room. If someone wants to feel bad because of not being there, that's a choice. *Not* being present may also be a beautiful expression of love. Many dying people are so attached to people they love that it's easier for them to die when those people aren't present. The energy of loved ones can hold us in a body we need to leave.

Perhaps you had to leave town before the actual death. That's OK. We are no less loving or loved because of where we are. We can tell the person before leaving that we love them and know they love us. A right expression of our love is to live the life we are given to live. Even if this never reaches spoken words, we know that **love is not expressed only by sitting at the bedside.**

A Practice Meditation for Leaving the Body

Knowing ahead of time what death *may* be like alleviates fear for some people. The following meditation may be useful *before* the actual time of death. At the moment of death, silence may be more appropriate. Read the meditation to yourself first. If it feels right in your heart ask if the dying person wants to try it. Sometimes it's clearly inappropriate.

It is not probable that a person will leave their body during the meditation, but it's possible. If the body dies, it's because it is time. Remember, the vehicle does not die until the soul decides to withdraw its energy. This meditation may be used as it is, or you may be inspired to create your own:

(The person's name), *we love you and we're ready to let you go. Feel a lighter body within your heavy physical body . . . move into your Light body. You don't need the old one anymore . . . Trust each moment . . . Let go of any distractions or anything that's holding you here. Softly and lightly. We're OK. God is within us and within you. God is in your heart. Surrender to who you are. Feel our love . . . God's love. We are love. If there is anything you haven't forgiven yourself for, forgive yourself now. (pause) We are One and we can never be separated . . . Move into the Light . . . Just keep moving into the clear Light . . . Nothing to hang on to . . .*

Whenever it feels right, just lift up and dissolve into the Light. There's no pain, only Light. Anything you see is a projection of your mind. Think God. See Light. 'Be not afraid for I am with you even in the shadow of death.' Move from the shadow into the Light . . . You will see and hear us. Don't be surprised if we can't hear you when it's your time to leave. The veil will not yet have lifted for us. You'll be met and welcomed on the other side and God will comfort us. You may review your life so that the lessons are clear . . . There is no punishment. Only unconditional love.

You're going Home . . . Home is the brightest Light. Move into the brightest Light. Know we love you and rejoice that you are God . . . You are free . . . Home to the one heart . . . total understanding . . . beauty . . . joy . . . We are One.

The Moment of Death

We use the phrase "moment of death" because that's how long death lasts. Just a moment.

The sound of silence may be the most loving gift right before the moment of death. At this moment, people of the Jewish faith say, *"Baruch Dayan ha-emet"* (Blessed is The

Judge of Truth); others say "Glory to God" or chant *"Om."* Others are silent.

At the moment of death the final thread holding the life force to the body releases. There is no pain. Consciousness leaves the dead body. I've seen the life force lift out of the body through the solar plexus, the heart, or the crown of the head. If you place your hand over these places at the moment of death, you may feel the energy going out. Your hand will tingle or feel different.

Immediately After Death

Do whatever is right for you. Be who you are. Be your heart. Share your hearts.

Thank God that this person you love is free.

> *Mother Father God, we ask that the Spirit of Living Love and Light be present to help* _____ *to his (her) new life..."*

Pray from your heart. Close your eyes and see what you see. Close your ears and hear what you hear.

Allow your tears, your grieving.

Breathe deeply, exhale deeply.

Hold someone who needs holding. Be held.

Hold the Light. Send your blessing with the newly free.

Send love to all around you.

Chant or sing a prayer.

Does anyone need extra help?

Make a circle holding hands and linking hearts.

Make a forgiveness circle: Each in turn in the words of each heart:

> *I forgive myself for each time in my life I have been less than loving with* _____ *(the one who's free). I forgive myself for each time in my life I have been less than loving with myself. I forgive myself for each time I have been less than loving with any of you. I accept my forgiveness. I accept your forgiveness. I accept that God has never judged me.*

Laying Out the Body

Treat the body with respect, knowing however that it's only a body. What you do with it in terms of cleaning and dressing has to do with your needs, not those of the new soul-being. Dressing the body is easier in the first hour, before it starts to stiffen. Unless you want to, it is not necessary to dress a body for cremation, for going to a hospital for examination or to a funeral home. We dressed Mary and John ourselves and didn't find it gruesome—just another task to be completed with love. Dad had promised the doctors at the VA hospital that they could examine his body so we didn't dress it.

In choosing clothes, think of what the person enjoyed wearing and how they'd like to be last seen. If a man was not a coat-and-tie type, it adds a jarring note to see him decked out like a Wall Street businessman or an attendant at someone else's funeral. It doesn't matter what some relatives or friends may think. They can do it their own way when it's their turn.

If it bothers you to see the eyes open, close them shortly after death. If the aesthetics of an open mouth bother you, tie a scarf around the head, like for a toothache, and leave it a few hours until the jaw sets closed.

After death, the body may involuntarily empty its bladder or bowels. Remember, it's a function of the body that is no longer related to the person. Personally I have not seen this and you may not either.

A short time after death, the faces of John, Mary and Dad looked more relaxed, peaceful and younger than while they were dying. All signs of the effort of leaving had gone.

There's no need to spend a lot of time with a body. Yet I recommend spending enough time with it so you really know it's only a cocoon. Go into the room where the body lies as often as feels right and perhaps talk with the soul, encouraging it to go free.

Getting a Death Certificate

To prevent legal complications, you'll need a death certificate signed by a physician or medical examiner. If a doctor is present at the death and has the certificate, he or she can sign it right away.

If a doctor is not present, call the one you've been working with. If you don't have one, call the medical examiner or county coroner. A doctor has to see the body before signing a death certificate. If it's in the middle of the night, wait until morning.

You will need copies of the death certificate for the state, bank(s), insurance companies, etc.

Advising Relatives and Friends

Advising relatives and friends of the death and burial plans should be done promptly because they may need time to get there. It's helpful to have a list with phone numbers and addresses ready. It could be a big help if someone volunteers to make the calls. However, if no one has had any sleep, all of this can wait until the next day. **Sleep!**

A Checklist of Things to Do

The checklist shared here is adapted from *A Manual of Death Education and Simple Burial* by Ernest Morgan. Some of these things need to be done shortly after the death and others may be done by you or friends in the weeks to come. Not all will apply to you or to your situation.
Take care of yourself first.

____ Decide on time and place of funeral or memorial services.
____ Make list of immediate family, close friends and employer or business colleagues. Notify each by phone.

___ If flowers are to be omitted, decide on appropriate memorial or charity to which gifts may be made.

___ Write obituary. Include age, place of birth, cause of death, occupation, college degrees, memberships held, military service, outstanding work, list of survivors in immediate family. Give time and place of memorial services. Deliver in person or by phone to newspapers.

___ Notify insurance companies, including automobile insurance for immediate cancellation and refund of premium.

___ Arrange for members of family or close friends to take turns answering door or phone, keeping careful record of calls.

___ Arrange appropriate child care.

___ Coordinate the supplying of food for the next days.

___ Consider special needs of the household, such as cleaning, etc., which might be done by friends.

___ Arrange hospitality for visiting relatives and friends.

___ Select pall bearers and notify. (Avoid men with heart or back difficulties, or make them honorary pall bearers.)

___ Notify lawyer and personal representative.

___ Plan for disposition of flowers after funeral (give to hospital or rest home?).

___ Prepare list of persons living at a distance to be notified by letter or printed notice, and decide which to send to each.

___ Prepare the message for printed notice if one is wanted.

___ Prepare list of persons to receive acknowledgements of flowers, calls, etc. Send appropriate acknowledgements. (May be written notes, printed acknowledgements, or some of each.)

___ Check carefully all life and casualty insurance policies and death benefits including Social Security, credit union, trade union, fraternal, military, etc. Check also on income for survivors from these sources.

___ Check promptly on all debts, mortgages, and installment payments. Some may carry life insurance clauses that will cancel the debt. If there is to be a delay in meeting payments, consult with creditors and ask for more time before the payments are due.

___ If deceased was living alone, notify utilities and landlord and tell post office where to send mail. Take precautions against thieves.

Bury me if you can catch me.
       —Socrates

Chapter 12

Planning a Burial and Service

A simple analogy for death that appeals to me is the butterfly leaving the cocoon. In a burial and memorial service, consider focusing on the beauty of the living butterfly instead of on the cocoon. Just as a butterfly doesn't need its discarded cocoon, a new soul-being doesn't need its old body.

If possible, make burial plans *ahead of time.* It may be more difficult to make practical decisions after the death than before. If you're feeling less than calm, you're more likely to let others—like the funeral industry, friends, clergy, etc.—take responsibility for arrangements. As we change our custom to *'It's not OK to profit by death',* there will be less worry about being victimized by an industry. If you can't make plans ahead, don't worry. You'll be surprised how everything will fall naturally into place.

Find out your state's law about how a body can be disposed of. Call the county coroner, State Board of Medical Examiners or a local memorial society (see page 231) for this information. In John's and Mary's cases all we knew ahead of time was that our state law permitted burial on private property.

When my dad was dying, we talked with him and without

him about plans, and my mother visited several funeral homes. I called the San Antonio city coroner to find out the Texas laws. Embalming wasn't legally required so we planned to have his body refrigerated, the coffin closed, and no visitors to the funeral home. My parents' home is in a little incorporated city within San Antonio so I also called the local courthouse. The chief of police said they had to come and investigate any death at home but because they knew my dad and what we planned, this wouldn't be necessary. A simple call avoided a police visit.

Let's look at the purposes of a burial service so you can create a meaningful one that nourishes you and fulfills the purpose.

1. To dispose of a cocoon.
2. To facilitate the process of grieving by allowing family and friends to express their love for the living spirit and for one another.

To Dispose of a Cocoon

Only when the earth shall claim your limbs, then shall you truly dance. —Kahlil Gibran

The choices for disposal of the body are cremation, burial or bequeathal to science. Find out what the dying person wants, and if possible, meet his or her wishes.

Unless you plan to bury the body yourself, I suggest you check first with a **memorial society.** A memorial society is a non-profit group of consumers who help members make pre-arrangements for a simple, economical burial. Because they're non-profit, they'll give you straight information about legal requirements, costs and arrangements. There are now about 200 memorial societies in the U.S. and Canada and more are springing up all the time. Look in the white pages of your telephone book under *Memorial Society* or *Funeral Society.* If you don't find a listing, see Appendix A, Useful

Addresses. Membership usually runs $10 to $25 and anyone can join. If you're quoted a higher membership price, it's probably not a real memorial society.

Some societies make arrangements for burials; some act as bargaining agents with funeral directors and make contracts for services; others simply provide information. In my experience they're fine people who know what's happening in the community and are very helpful. Ernest Morgan's excellent booklet, *A Manual of Death Education and Simple Burial,* is available from memorial societies.

CREMATION

Burning a body until only ashes remain is a clean, simple, economical way of returning earth to earth. Actual cremation costs are $125 to $200. Services such as picking up the body and doing the paperwork are additional costs. For example, one group in San Antonio does the whole job for $325. You can take the body to a crematorium (sometimes called a crematory) yourself or have it taken to a funeral home for cremation.

Most crematoriums require a 'suitable container' for transporting the body and will sell you a cardboard box. Some crematories will accept a body on a stretcher. After the cremation, you can keep or scatter the ashes in a meaningful place. Indiana is the only state that prohibits scattering ashes. A niche for the ashes in a cemetery may cost $150 to $300 or more.

I've heard medical examiners say we're moving toward cremation as the preferred method of disposal in the U.S. as the population is increasing and land prices are rising.

EARTH BURIAL

This has become extremely costly unless you live in a state that permits burial on private property or the person is eligible to be buried in a National Cemetery (see page 81 for eligibility).

If your state permits burial on private property, it can be very satisfying to do the burial yourself. *Plan ahead.* You will need to present the death certificate to the local registrar of vital statistics to obtain a burial or transit permit. A professional carpenter or friend can build the coffin. For an adult, the box should be six inches to one foot longer than the person, about one to one and a half feet deep, and two feet to three feet wide. It should have a separate top that can be put on later. Line the box and decorate the outside if you wish. Use the box to transport the body to the chosen burial place, where you'll probably want to have a service. For digging, you will need shovels and picks.

Home burials cost almost nothing. John's burial cost $150. This included two trees to start the orchard and food and drink for the celebration. Friends donated the wood for the coffin and built it. Mary's funeral cost $44, which included wood for the coffin, gasoline for two trucks and beer to refresh the diggers.

If the laws in your state don't permit burial on private property or you don't want to handle the arrangements yourself, there are several alternatives: the non-profit memorial societies already mentioned, reasonable-profit memorial *services* and traditional funeral homes.

MEMORIAL SERVICES

These are profit-making groups which bury bodies at reasonable prices. For example, the San Antonio group does a $300 pine coffin service (not including interment fees). It was started by a friendly dentist/undertaker who paid his way through dental school doing embalming, got disgusted with what he saw in the funeral industry, and decided to start something new. There are a number of similar services in California and Florida and there'll be many more. Like funeral homes, memorial services pick up the body, take care of legal procedures and paperwork (such as permits, VA and Social Security benefits), and handle arrangements. A memorial or funeral *society* can tell you if there's a reasonably priced memorial service in your area, or you can look in the Yellow Pages under *Funerals* and call to check prices.

FUNERAL HOMES

Traditional funeral homes may soon be on their way out unless they change to meet people's needs at reasonable prices. They're the only ones who do embalming and cosmetic work and they're responsible for some state laws that say a person can't be buried unless they're embalmed. If a funeral director tells you embalming is necessary, check with the medical examiner or county coroner. *In most places embalming is **not** a legal requirement.*

The alternatives to embalming are to dispose of the body within 24 hours or to refrigerate it until the service. To rationalize embalming, funeral directors have said that it's an important aid to the grieving process, that families need to view the body. It's true that viewing the body is important; it seems to cauterize the emotional wound. Even in the event of sudden death, the body may be viewed on the spot or in the emergency room of a hospital. In a home death you've had time to experience the physical reality of death and there's usually no need for 'viewing the body'.

If you use a funeral home, get an itemized list of costs in writing *ahead of time.* They sometimes neglect to tell you all the costs and you receive a much bigger bill than you'd expected.

Don't believe anyone who tells you a $150 casket doesn't show the respect of a $2,000 one. *Respect is an attitude, not a coffin.* The dying person may have already expressed definite ideas and preferences on this subject.

A fancy coffin is not an effective way to deal with either grief or guilt. If you like a big show, why not have a super party? Why finance a funeral director's party? Or, you might want to give the money you'd have spent to a group or a person who needs it, perhaps one favored by the person who died.

The Department of Commerce reported that in 1977, the most recent year for which they had figures, the average funeral cost through a funeral home was $2400, *not* including plot and interment which could easily bring the total to over $3000. My dad's funeral in 1981 cost $1455. Of this, my mom paid $800, Social Security $255 and VA $400. It was a very simple funeral. If my dad hadn't been eligible for burial in a National Cemetery, all of it would have cost about $2500.

Cemetery space is expensive. In Santa Fe, for example, a ground burial now costs $710 ($265 for the plot, $100 for perpetual care, $200 for a vault—a moisture resistant casket cover— and $145 for opening and closing the grave). And this is considered a real steal. In larger cities, costs are generally higher. One Albuquerque cemetery charges $1,200 for a plot.

BEQUEATHAL OF THE BODY

Bequeathal of the body or parts of it to science is another way to dispose of a cocoon (see page 204). If the person has signed a Uniform Donor's Card, find it and call the closest medical school. Some schools have more bodies than they need, others not enough. They'll generally pick up the body. If you live at a great distance from the school, however, you may have to pay for part of the transportation costs. Ask them while you're on the phone. Included in the release form is what you want done with the body after it has served its usefulness to the medical profession.

Rituals and Celebrations

A ritual or celebration facilitates the process of grieving by allowing family and friends to express their love for the living spirit and for each other.

Leaving a physical vehicle (the body) is an important rite of passage both for the person doing it and for the family and friends. A ritual marking this change helps us express our sadness and loss with others before we face the changed reality without the person's physical presence.

The ritual you create can be a celebration of life. We can celebrate the life completed, and through it, all of life. We can celebrate Love. We can celebrate having been fortunate enough to share time together. We can share love and support for each other. The celebration can also help us express our grief, sadness, and perhaps anger that we're left to take care of daily business.

Jewish *shivas,* Irish and Polish wakes, and Hispanic *veladas* (candlelight watches) have long been useful forms for exploring and sharing loss and renewing old relationships.

You might use an old form or create a new one. Allow a ritual or celebration to grow in whatever way feels appropriate for you. Choose a place that's meaningful—indoors or out in nature. Does it matter if the body is present or not? Do you, the people involved, want to speak about your feelings for the person? Would you rather be silent? Do you want someone to lead the ceremony or can each person share in their own way? Do you want clergy or do you want to be your own ministers and celebrants? Do you want flowers, music, poetry? Do you want to share food together or dancing or song? What about a prayer circle, a hugging or holding circle? Even digging can be part of the ritual. You may want to use the 'Forgiveness Circle' (page 225). The possibilities are infinite.

In a ritual, I believe we need to focus on releasing the soul even if it is difficult for us. If we cling to it, the soul's love for us can make it difficult for it to move away from family, friends and the familiar physical world and on to its new life. We're accustomed to thinking there is nothing further we can do for someone after she or he dies. We speak at our services as if they weren't there. I believe they are there and that we can still help. We can talk with the person, let them know we're

OK and encourage them to go free. We can offer prayers of thanksgiving for life that never ends and we can *continue* to share our hearts.

Working with Clergy

If your spiritual understanding and practices have been related to a particular religious group, you may want to ask your minister, rabbi or priest for help in planning a service. The clergy have shared their knowledge and compassion many times with dying people and their families. They do have a commitment to do things in the manner prescribed by their particular faith. Check within yourself to see if their suggestions meet the earlier wishes of the person as well as your own sense of rightness. Everyone has equal access to God.

What to Wear

"Darn, I don't have a black dress or suit. Will navy blue do?"

What to wear for a funeral is still an issue for many people.

Some people don't have black clothing because they don't like black. It makes me feel locked in, constricted, as though I can't express myself. Wearing black forms a shield around the body that retards energy going in or out and protects us when we're emotionally weak. But the price of this protection is high. Black locks in energy, including sadness, grief and love. In countries where it's the custom to wear black for a long mourning period, holding in feelings frequently becomes a way of life. In my view, wearing black is like a heavy casket—it keeps things in. Can you remember anyone wearing black in all those paintings of the death of Christ? No, they wore white or light colors. White is expansive and reflects energy. As light, it includes all colors. Wear a color you like or one you know the butterfly liked.

We can reflect the rainbow. Respect is an attitude, not a color.

A Life Celebration to Share Later

The blessing you've felt in having shared time and love with someone doesn't end just because they're no longer here in a body.

In the months to come, you might want to create something to celebrate their life... and your life: a garden, an orchard, a carved cross, or whatever. Making a card or writing a story or poem can be a healing way to share someone's movement from life to life, particularly with friends who weren't present for the death or burial.

Many people expect the anniversary of physical death or the person's birthday to be a day of sadness. We can make them days to celebrate as well. Months after John died a friend hauled a rock off a mesa, carved it and set it on John's grave. The card shown here is about a man I never knew.

Allen Morgan Parrott
November 5, 1918 – January 11, 1979

It is eternity now.
I am in the midst of it.
It is about me in the sunshine;
I am in it,
as the butterfly in the light-laden air.
Nothing has to come;
it is now.
Now is eternity;
now is the immortal life.

Richard Jefferies

Allen Parrott

If anyone understood the hidden rhythms of growth,
                    Allen did.

He was a good gardener,
with his full share of a gardener's sensibilities.

One sometimes felt that he was more comfortable
communing with plants than with people.
. . . At least he never seemed to draw that arbitrary line
between the animate and inanimate in terms of talk.
A flower has its own dialect, and he could accept that.

Farm boy gone to Berkeley, he discovered how to link
literature, philosophy and art with the sun and soil,
weaving fruit and flower into harmonies of hand-dyed wool.
(No intellectual phoniness here. He knew where the real source lay:
outdoors, not in.)

Loving husband, father, friend, he was all of these,
and therefore missed.
But that's our problem now, not his . . .

for beyond the too specific limits of physical frailty
and tick-tock time, that sometimes made him crotchety,

if anyone ever enjoyed the inexpressible range
of boundless freedom,
                    Allen does.

A card for Allen Parrott

Weeping may endure for a night, but joy cometh in the morning.

Psalms 30:5

Chapter 13

Grieving

*Perhaps the most important reason for 'lamenting' is
that it helps us to realize our oneness with all things, to
know that all things are our relatives...*
                                                —Black Elk

If you know in your heart that your loved one is alive,
although alive in a different way, you may feel joy as well as
sadness. Allow joy. Allow relief. If your relationship with the
person wasn't central to your life, you probably won't feel
sad. That's fine. No need to pretend to grieve. But if you do
feel pain, you need to express it so you don't suffer later.

Allow yourself your grieving. Allow it to express in whatever way feels right to you. Grieving is the way we heal the
loss we feel for someone we love. You're not crazy; a deep
bursting sorrow is one reflection of the *value* in your life of
this close relationship that has changed form. You may have
feelings similar to those the person had while dying: denial,
isolation, guilt, anger, bargaining, depression and acceptance.

Cry those oceans if they're there. Yell. Be sad, be lonely,
be angry. Move your body. Don't let anyone tell you to be

quieter—they can do it their way when it's their turn to grieve. Yell at "John the Bastard" for leaving you. Yell at "God the Merciless" for taking your loved one away. God can take it. Let it spill out from all the nooks and crannies of your being. Cry all those things you didn't cry about in the past. Clean out old sadness.

At one time or another the emptiness comes. Know this space. It may be with you for a time and it may be one of the most important spaces in your life. It's in this quiet after the outward grieving that the seeds for your new life begin to grow. Some people call this emptiness the 'Dark Night of the Soul'. You've let go of something precious and familiar and the new meaning is not yet known. It takes a lot of courage to be alive in this emptiness. Just be with it. Pay attention to what is trying to grow . . . new qualities or ways of being, new ideas about work, whatever.

There is an old Zen saying, *"You can't fill a teacup that is already full."* If we allow the emptiness, we can move to a new fullness.

As you begin to understand what is trying to grow, and if you're willing, make it a choice to nourish these tiny seedlings. If you panic, you may stomp down little new beginnings. A lot of people panic. I have. Because this emptiness can be unknown and frightening, people often rush to fill the void with busy-ness or suffering—perhaps the closest, most familiar thing at this moment. Maybe we say to ourselves, *'Better to feel something, even if it's suffering, than nothing.'* It's true a vacuum looks to be filled. And we have a choice of what *we* fill it with. We have a *choice!* You can use this quiet space instead of it using you. Catch up on sleep, pray, meditate, take long walks, work with the earth . . . prepare your soil.

When our hearts break, they break open, making more room for everybody and everything, more love, more joy, more compassion. We can stay open to the loneliness and pain, knowing it is moving us to a new fullness. Or we can shut down. A heart that has broken open, doesn't close unless we close it. We have free will to close it or let it stay open.

Part of grieving is fear. We're afraid we've lost our love, that somehow it's gone with the physical body of the person. Without the soul that shone through the body or personality of that person we probably wouldn't have loved him or her in the first place. And that soul is not gone. We don't have to stop thinking about or loving the person, although in time that love moves to another place in our being. I believe it is inaccurate to assume that the *object* of our love *is* our love. We *are* love, so we can never lose it. Your love is present even while you're grieving.

Give *your* love to yourself. When you're able, give it to the people around you. If there aren't any, find new people and situations where you can share love. When you give it away it returns to you increased. There can never be too much, and it will nourish everyone you meet. If we don't express our feelings, including the love we are, we will feel depressed. Our love backs up on us. I don't remember having felt depressed around people I love while they were dying. The depression comes afterward, when suddenly there's no longer a focus for all that energy . . . no one to care for . . . no clear way of expressing love. The solution is to look for new ways to express the love . . . not too difficult really. It's needed everywhere.

I see two kinds of grieving: grieving for cleansing and purification and grieving as a habit of suffering that hasn't been replaced with something more nourishing. One is an essential step in growth and the other offers no movement. Treading water. Who wants to tread water the rest of their lives? It's tiring . . . and boring. Cleansing and purification provide space for new growth that may be very exciting.

If you feel stuck in suffering, get help. Find a friend or a counselor. Someone who works with Gestalt or other techniques that focus on releasing stuck feelings may be useful. Some cultures have met the need for grieving with wailing, dancing, chanting—all ways of releasing pent-up energies.

However, many people in our culture find such releases embarrassing, so sometimes we may need counselors. People probably won't need them anymore when they stop making judgements against expressing their feelings, appreciating instead the help that expressing feelings can give in adjusting to life's great changes.

If you're alone at home and have already let out the tears and the pain still feels too heavy, send love to the *part of you* that feels it. Try compressing time. Imagine yourself a year from now: How are you feeling? Is there now more space around the pain? Write your feelings on paper. Talk, perhaps out loud, to the person who's gone. She or he can hear you. Dr. Moody and Dr. Kübler-Ross, and others, confirm this.

During your grieving, allow friends the opportunity to share with you. Lots of people are skilled givers and not so skilled as receivers. Let friends have the joy of giving. They'll feel privileged that you chose to talk with them about your feelings and the person you love. Sometimes they may help you recognize the new seeds sprouting. And they can hold you when you need it. Know that friends want to share their love but some may not know how. Tell them what you need. Often it's after the first month, when the shock and numbness are wearing off, that we particularly need their support.

In the jungles of Mexico one custom after someone dies is that each person who comes to the burial or to visit asks the mourner to recount the story of how the death happened. The visitors probably already know, but the point is to keep the mourner repeating and repeating the story until the shock lessens and he or she begins to accept what's happened. Friends can do the same thing for us . . . listen and listen and listen. Share your story.

If a child is mourning the loss of a parent, I highly recommend Eda LeShan's *Learning to Say Goodbye*. It's a loving, sensitive book an older child (9-10) can read to him or herself, or which a remaining parent or child may benefit from sharing. A teenager or an adult might feel less alone after reading Dorothy Maclean's *To Hear the Angels Sing*. If you can't find it in a bookstore, you can order it from Findhorn Publications in Scotland (see Appendix H).

Another helpful book is Harriet Sarnoff Schiff's *The Bereaved Parent,* published by Penquin Books.

And take time to appreciate yourself. You are the same person who began this experience—and something more.

WHAT WE CAN DO FOR LOVED ONES
IS
LOVE OURSELVES

And let us, above all things, never forget that in due course the dead will come back, and we never know when we shall see looking out at us from the eyes of a little child a soul we have known. Let us therefore, making expression for the love that now may have no earthly outlet, turn it to the endeavor of making the world a better place for the return of those we love.

—Dion Fortune
Through the Gates of Death

Chapter 14

Life After Death

People sleep and when they die they awake.
—Mohammad

Your own heart is the source of knowing about life after death.

I can share with you my reality and how I arrived at it. I can tell you about recent studies and writings across the ages. All these are just footnotes to your own knowing.

If you're willing, try this:

Find a quiet place and close your eyes. Breathe gently inside and let go of any ideas you have about life after death. Become 'empty'. If thoughts come up, don't get caught up in them . . . just watch them. Breathe into your heart and from this place ask for guidance . . . Ask if death exists other than as a change in form. Ask if you are born again and again. **Trust** *what you hear, especially if it is a calm and gentle inner voice. If nothing comes, trust that this is OK too.*

My own sense is that life after death and rebirth are two of the best-kept secrets in the West. Working with dying people I've found that most have had hints or visions that life continues, and/or that they have lived before. Many shared experiences that they had not shared before for fear of being ridiculed. When they felt that I wouldn't judge them crazy or senile, they felt free to talk. We learn a lot more about our human experience when people feel free to share their experiences without fear of being judged.

Elisabeth Kübler-Ross has said, "I don't have a shadow of doubt death (as an end) doesn't really exist... If they hang me up by my toes I won't stop exploring life after death."

Raymond Moody, M.D., in his popular book *Life After Life,* reports the experiences of people who 'officially died' and were resuscitated. Since his book appeared, numerous books and articles have been published by medical doctors who received firsthand reports from patients and by people who have had the experience themselves.

What Dr. Moody reports basically agrees with what patients have told me and what I've read in other doctors' reports, in books, recent newspaper articles and the *Brain Mind Bulletin.* From his interviews with people who died and were resuscitated, Dr. Moody reported:

1. When the 'officially dead' persons heard someone say they were dead, they felt afraid and surprised and wanted to be back in their bodies.
2. After the initial fear, they felt incredibly peaceful.
3. Some reported hearing noises, buzzing, ringing, roaring, chimes or bells.
4. Most experienced a dark space, often described as a tunnel, which they moved through quickly.
5. Many then experienced being outside of their bodies and looking down, surprised at the efforts being made to revive them. Seeing and vision seemed enhanced.
6. Most reported reunions with friends and relatives who had died earlier, a sort of greeting committee.
7. Nearly all experienced a beautiful luminous light or a *light being* who felt enormously loving. The identification of this *light being* was determined by their experience before

death. (Dr. Karlis Osis and Erlendur Haraldsson made a cross-cultural study between the U.S. and India and found that Christians interpreted the *light being* as Christ and Hindus interpreted it as a Hindu diety. Both Asians and Americans saw the dark passage, brilliant light and dead relatives.)

8. The *light being* often suggested that the person review their life. No one reported feeling this was punitive, only instructive.

9. The person then reached a barrier or limit where they felt they must make a choice whether or not to return to life. Most found *being dead* so beautiful that returning was a hard decision. Many decided to return because of their children and spouses.

10. After the experience, most felt they would not be afraid to die again. And their experience of life was enhanced.

What about hell? I don't believe there is a literal hell. I agree with Elisabeth Kübler-Ross, "Hell is just what we do to each other." Hell is punishment. If life is a school for remembering we are love, would God punish people because we stumble or fall? Seems unlikely to me. I imagine that each time we fall, the God part of us picks us up, dusts us off, says "I love you," and we start again. No one punishes us except ourselves. Evidently after we die, we review our lives so we are aware of and can learn from our experiences. Perhaps this review is what some have called hell or purgatory. It could indeed be pretty awful to reexperience some of the unloving things we've done. We don't have to continue doing these things by withholding love from ourselves and others.

What about sin and evil? To me they are energy we haven't looked into deeply enough to understand. Sin and evil are a lack of love, and so we are healed by love, not punishment. At times we may have to physically segregate a person so they won't hurt us, and to give them a chance to learn love. Prisons won't be effective deterrents until they teach love.

In his book, *Beyond Death's Door* Maurice Rawlings, M.D. reports studies similar to Dr. Moody's. Some of his patients reported unpleasant experiences when they 'died' and he interprets them as possibly representing hell. I feel they represented a person's own negative projections. We project something dreadful to teach us about love while we can still return and make changes in our lives. Remember Ebenezer Scrooge's experience in Dicken's *A Christmas Carol?*

We get what we expect. If we expect a hell, we may get one!

Punishment is a form of manipulation. Perhaps hell was invented so some groups could control their members with fear. Many organized religions suggest that their way is the only way to God. Follow instructions or be punished! This is not to deny the beauty of organized religions, but only to point out that they are made up of human beings like ourselves who have free will and are, therefore, fallible.

I believe we can't give the responsibility for our relationship with God to someone else. We are each responsible for this relationship.

Until the Second Council of Constantinople in A.D. 553, presided over by the Emperor Augustinian, reincarnation, which teaches that we are responsible, was in the Bible. For more than 500 years, reincarnation, "the mystical doctrine," was widely accepted by Christians, including the most eminent church fathers. The council declared it heresy, called it the *"mythical* doctrine" and deleted it after a 3 to 2 vote. Perhaps it was in the 'best interests' of the Church for people not to know they had more than one chance to get to heaven or that eventually everyone gets there no matter what their religious path.* Reincarnation is still found in the writings of St.

---

* The edict of the Second Council of Constantinople said: "Whosoever shall support the mythical doctrine of the preexistence of the soul and the consequent wonderful opinion of its return, let him be anathema." Pope Vigilius never authorized the "anathema," but it was generally believed that he had. Since the Church has never made an *official* statement against reincarnation it's perhaps possible for a practicing Catholic to believe in reincarnation without being in technical disagreement with Church doctrine.

Augustine, who inspires Catholics and non-Catholics alike.

Reincarnation's teaching is that everyone is in the process of going home to God or growing to godhood, and we are born again and again until we reach that perfection. Each soul is created equal to every other soul and has free will to remember it is love in its own way and time. *No time or way is 'better' than another.* The paths home are as many as the people on the planet. Nothing can stop us, although we may experience what some call delays. Delays are opportunities to deepen our understanding.

Reincarnation teaches that we choose when and to whom we will be born. We choose our parents, the ones most suitable to provide the environment we need to complete any un-learned lessons. As a soul, we enter the physical child con-ceived by the chosen parents. We reincarnate in groups, so we see again and again people we've loved and helped as well as ones we've hated and hurt. It's no accident that we come together as families and friends to learn.

We also choose when we will die. When the soul sees that the body is no longer in condition to continue learning and remembering, it gives a signal for the dying process to begin. Sometimes the soul leaves the body before the body stops functioning. This may explain a feeling that many people re-port: they're with someone who is near death and sense that the person is *not there.*

Reincarnation includes the teaching that here on earth we create, allow or tolerate everything we experience in order to help us learn and remember. No one is really a victim. Assuming that we are victims is a way people have avoided taking responsibility for being co-creators. Once we remember who we really are and become responsible co-creators, we don't need to be born again unless we choose to in order to serve our fellow human beings.

'Whatsoever a man sows, that shall he also reap' (Galatians 6:7). Women too! The cause and effect of our actions is sometimes called the *Law of Karma.* The law is a description of how energy works. Plant a carrot seed, reap a carrot. Give love, receive love. Karma may also be understood as the *judgements* we make that keep us feeling separate and as all our *unlearned lessons.*

Karma means we're responsible and accountable for all past choices and actions, *no matter how small;* we reap the blessings and the teachings. Being sick, having a car accident or going to jail are not punishments or 'bad karma'. They're opportunities *we've created* to help us remember and learn, so we can change our lives and live with more joy now.

There is also *group karma.* I believe, for example, it's the karma of the human race and individuals to learn unity. World War II had to do with group karma, but no one chose to be born into that time who didn't have the *individual* karma to learn from the experience.

Unconditional love *doesn't* create Karma. If in any action love was my intention, I'm responsible for love. If hate was my intention, I'm responsible for that hate, and karma is created. 'Working out karma'—being responsible for what we feel, think and do—teaches love and compassion and helps us move beyond separation to awareness of unity.

Unconditional love transcends karma. (Divine will transcends the cause and effect of human will.) Sometimes this is called the *Law of Grace.* It's the teaching of *compassion* that Jesus Christ added to older teachings of divine justice. (karma).

If one becomes a different person from the one who created the karma (by repenting, rethinking, changing, transforming), then she or he is free of it. Justice is the great teaching of the mind; compassion and freedom are teachings of the heart.

If we choose, we can break the cycle of birth, death and rebirth by loving unconditionally. When we live love, we live the truth of unity and no longer the illusion of separation. There are no more unlearned lessons. We know that everything is equally sacred and see God in everything, no matter how disguised the form. We're free.

It may take many lifetimes to live the unconditional love that we are *and* it's possible for each of us to live it this lifetime, right now.

*No man is an island . . . (each) is a piece of the continent, a
part of the main . . ."* —John Donne*

In a very real sense, helping someone else see the God
within is helping ourselves. Not until the last lamb is home are
we all really home. Our work is to Love, Serve and Remember.

When we see all of nature working in cycles, I often wonder
why we don't envision the same for ourselves. Is it arrogance or
is it fear that we'll lose our individuality, our specialness, if we're
part of the whole? Are we confusing uniformity with unity?
Each flower, tree, sunset and human being is a unique expression of the whole. We see a seed planted, growing to maturity,
bearing fruit and releasing seeds that sprout anew. Over and
over we see the cycles of birth and death and rebirth. Are we
not part of the cyclical process of nature as well? *Does not the
seed-core in us go on to a new period of growth after we drop
our bodies?*

*   *   *

I'd like to share with you how my understanding of the
continuity of life grew. As a child, when I was still closely
connected to my heart-knowing, I knew that life didn't end. But
everyone said it ended with death and they were bigger than
me, and I wanted their approval. (Interestingly, Dr. Kübler-
Ross reports that children up to five years old believe death is
reversible.) It didn't make sense to me that we came into the
world and did this little dance and were snuffed out.

I heard a lot of talk about justice, loving our brothers, freedom and perfection that didn't make sense in terms of what I
saw. "Why are they starving?" "Why was their son killed in an
accident?" "Why are we so lucky?" "Why does his wife treat

---

*John Donne wrote in 1623: "No man is an island, entire of itself; every man is a piece
of the continent, a part of the main; if a clod be washed away by the sea, Europe is the
less, as well as if a promontory were, as well as if a manor of thy friends or of thine
own were; any man's death diminishes me, because I am involved in mankind; and
therefore never send to know for whom the bell tolls; it tolls for thee."

him so badly?'' ''Why is she dying of cancer?—she lived such a good life.''

It seems unfair! It looks like chaos!

Then I noticed there were some things I really loved and some I hated and most of the time I didn't know why. For a while, I loved everything Black American, Native American, Persian and Tibetan and hated everything German. I didn't think I was a racist . . . so why hate Germans? Out of ten years living in Europe, I spent *one night* in Germany. That night I was so terrified that I barricaded my hotel room door with a dresser and chairs. Definitely not rational!

First with the help of friends guiding me and then alone, I slowly began to remember past lives.

I *remembered* having been a German Jew who died at Büchenwald. After I remembered, I began to understand. I was judging the Germans as they had judged me. They made Jews separate. I made Germans separate. There is a 'Hitler' in me—the part of me that judges. I forgave myself for making that separation and now love Germans as I would anyone else. There is a 'Hitler' in each of us. It's the part that separates us from each other and unity.

The Jews and Germans sacrificed to give us another chance to remember *we are love*. Will we listen to the gentle teaching of love, or will we create something horrible to remind us again? It's our choice.

Gradually I have begun to experience life's energy as a wave manifesting into form and dissolving into formlessness. Justice and all those beautiful ideas make sense if we are moving toward manifesting them over a number of lives. I began to see that what I'd interpreted as chaos were opportunities to learn. I *know again* in my heart that death is just a word we invented to describe letting go of a shell. Life is endless . . . only the form changes.

APPENDIX A

Useful Addresses

Cancer Counseling and Research Center

This center does counseling based on the work of Dr. Carl Simonton and Stephanie M. Simonton. The Simontons have combined meditation, progressive relaxation and visual imagery in treating cancer. Taped materials are available.

Cancer Counseling and Research Center
P.O. Box 1055
Azle, TX 76020
Telephone: 817-444-4073

Color Therapy

They provide written consultation and a series of color treatments. Write for costs. They send color healing to you over a period of time. If it's an emergency, let them know.

Secretary, White Lodge
Stockland Green Road, Speldhurst
Nr. Tunbridge Wells, Kent, TN3 OT7
England
Telephone: 0892-86-3166

Concern for Dying

Concern for Dying is an educational council that publishes a newsletter and will send you a Living Will form. Their address is the same as the Society for the Right to Die.

Concern for Dying
250 West 57th Street
New York, NY 10019
(212) 246-6962

Shanti Nilaya

This center founded by Elisabeth Kubler-Ross holds regular retreats for dying patients, their families, and professionals in the field. (For the "Dougy Letter" send $2.95.)

Shanti Nilaya
Star Route A - Box 28
Headwaters, VA 24442

Silent Unity

Silent Unity is a group in Missouri who will pray for anyone, for whatever is the highest good. When you call in a name, yours or anyone else's, it is taken to a Room of Light for 30 days. Someone remains in the room 24 hours a day, praying for these people.

Silent Unity
Unity Village, MO 64065
(816) 524-3550
(800) 821-2935 (toll free)

Society for the Right to Die

The Society works for the recognition of the individual's right to die with dignity. Write to them for Living Will Declarations and the appropriate documents authorized by right-to-die laws and other related material.

Society for the Right to Die
250 W. 57th Street
New York, NY 10107
(212) 246-6973

Southwestern College of Life Sciences

This college offers degrees in transformational counseling and seminars in working with different levels of consciousness. I studied with them for years and found their work excellent. If enough people want to take it, you can arrange for a workshop in your area.

Southwestern College of Life Sciences
209 MacKenzie Street
Santa Fe, NM 87501
(505) 982-1805

The following organizations have groups or centers across the country, Canada and Europe. Check your local phone book or contact the offices listed below for the group nearest you.

Funeral and Memorial Societies

Many thoughtful people in the U.S. and Canada have found membership in a memorial society the best way to assure dignity, simplicity and economy in funeral arrangements. Advance planning through a society also avoids stressful and costly decisions at time of death.

Look in the white pages of your phone book under "Funeral Societies" or "Memorial Socities" or contact The Continental Association to find the Society nearest you.

The Continental Association
   of Funeral & Memorial Societies
2001 S Street, N.W., Suite 530
Washington, DC 20009

               or

The Memorial Society Association of Canada
Box 96, Station "A"
Weston, Ontario M9N 3M6

Hospices

There are now over 1200 existing or developing hospices in the U.S. and Canada giving care to terminally ill patients and their families. Call your local hospital, visiting nurse service, or contact the National Hospice Organization to find out if there is one near you.

National Hospice Organization
1901 No. Ft. Myer Drive
Arlington, VA 22209
Telephone: (703) 243-5900

Uniform Donor Card Sources

Copies of the Uniform Donor's Card are available free of charge through:

American Medical Association
535 North Dearborn Street
Chicago, IL 60610
Attention: Order Department

Eye-Bank Association of America
1111 Tulane Avenue
New Orleans, LA 70112

Living Bank
Hermann Professional Building, Suite 818
Houston, TX 77005

Medic Alert
P.O. Box 1009
Turlock, CA 95380

National Pituitary Agency
Suite 503-7
210 West Fayette Street
Baltimore, MD 21201

National Kidney Foundation
116 East 27th Street
New York, NY 10016

APPENDIX B

The Bach Flower Remedies

The basic cause of disease is due to disharmony between the personality and the Soul. The Bach Remedies help restore that harmony.
—Dr. Edward Bach (1886-1936)

There are a number of ways to determine which flowers are needed. The simplest way, unless you know how to use a pendulum, is to talk with the person you're diagnosing. Then, using what she or he says and your own intuition, choose from the list below. If you use a pendulum, place the flower bottles close to the person, inside their auric field, and select the flowers that swing 'positive'.

To mix remedies use a ½ oz. or 1 oz. brown dropper bottle, fill it with spring water and add ¼ dropper of brandy. Add two drops from the stock flower bottles you've selected. Then shake the bottle 50 times. For chronic problems take about ¼ dropperful four times a day. For acute problems or crises, take a few drops every 10 or 15 minutes. You can also add drops to juice or water, bath water and massage lotions. Use in combinations of up to five remedies.

Rescue Remedy is a premixed composite remedy for all emergencies or crisis situations. It's composed of Star of Bethlehem, Rock Rose, Impatiens, Cherry Plumb and Clematis.

To order remedies, write:

The Secretary
The Dr. Edward Bach Centre
Mounternon, Sotwill
Wallingfor, Oxon
OX10 OPZ, England

The flowers cost approximately $38.00 and will last about ten years with regular use.

For those who have fear:

ROCK ROSE: For terror, panic, extreme fright. Give to the patient and to the people around him or her. Fear is conquered by a state of mind wherein the "small self" is forgotten in the need of the moment. Great courage, daring and compassion are the antidote for fear.

MIMULUS: For fear or anxiety of a known origin. Fears of everyday life. "All fear must be cast out: it should never exist in the human mind, and is only possible when we lose sight of our Divinity." Positive qualities: understanding, courage, humor.

CHERRY PLUM: Desperation, fear of losing one's mind or of doing something dreadful. The positive Cherry Plum person has quiet, calm courage and endurance under stress.

ASPEN: Fears of unknown origin. Unexplained feeling of anxiety. Low pain threshold. The opposite virtue to cultivate is "fearlessness because of the knowledge that the universal power of love stands behind all. It makes the desire to invite experience and adventure because we know we can walk thru any danger unafraid."

RED CHESTNUT: Excessive fear and anxiety for others, especially those dear to us. Anticipating misfortune for others. Positive quality is the ability to send out thoughts of safety, health or courage to those who need them, especially if they're in danger or ill.

For those who suffer uncertainty:

CERATO: Distrust of self, doubt, foolishness, talkativeness. Saps other's vitality. Positive qualities: Quiet assurance, intuitive, sure of ability and judgment.

SCLERANTHUS: Undecided between two choices; imbalance. Difficulty in concentrating. Positive qualities: Calm, decisive people, poised and balanced.

GENTIAN: Doubt, depression and discouragement from a known cause. Failure, negative attitude. Positive qualities: Individuals who never let anything get them down. No failure when doing your best.

GORSE: Hopelessness, despair. "They are generally sallow and rather dark of complexion, often with dark lines beneath their eyes . . . Need sunshine to drive the clouds away." Strength may be gained in acceptance of suffering. Positive qualities: faith, hope.

HORNBEAM: Tiredness, weariness, mental and physical exhaustion. Auric contamination. Learn to coordinate time with effort, taking advantage of energy cycles and to use the energy of joy.

WILD OAT: Uncertainty in talented people who can't determine their course in life. Discovery of the Soul's purpose gives life direction. "If a case suggests that it needs many Remedies, or if the person does not respond to treatment, give either *Holly* or *Wild Oat,* and it will then be obvious which other Remedies may be required."

Not sufficient interest in present circumstances:

CLEMATIS: Dreamy, bored, unconscious, absent-minded, sensitive, mediumistic, poor memory. Positive qualities: Sensitive to inspiration and guidance from dreams. People who take a lively interest.

HONEYSUCKLE: Nostalgia, homesickness, dwelling upon thoughts of the past too much. Being able to use the past, with its emotional memories, but also being able to live now.

OLD ROSE: Resignation, apathy, passivity, boredom. "Let us turn life into an adventure of absorbing interest. . . ." The joy of gaining experience and helping others.

OLIVE: Complete exhaustion, total fatigue of mind and body, especially after a long illness. Restores vitality, strength and an interest in life. Learn to pace yourself.

WHITE CHESTNUT: Persistent unwanted thoughts; mental arguments and conversations. Knows how to control thought and imagination and can use them creatively. Useful for sleeplessness.

MUSTARD: Black depression, gloom. "This Remedy dispels gloom and brings joy into life."

CHESTNUT BUD: Failure to learn by experience, hence repetition. Lack of observation. "This Remedy is to help us take full advantage of our daily experiences, and to see ourselves and our mistakes as others do." Keen observation, able to balance opposites.

Loneliness:

WATER VIOLET: Quiet, self-reliant people who are proud and aloof. Stiffness in mind and body. Positive: "Those who have great gentleness, are tranquil, sympathetic, wise, practical counselors, who have poise and dignity and pass gracefully through life."

IMPATIENS: Impatience, irritability, extreme mental tension. Makes quick decisions. For people quick in mind and action who can become exhausted through frustration when things don't move fast enough. Positive: Gentle and sympathetic, tolerant, considerate.

HEATHER: Self-centered, self-concerned, talks constantly. Saps others' energy. Understanding person who has suffered much and is willing to listen to and help others.

Over-sensitive to influences and ideas:

AGRIMONY: Mental torture, worry and fear concealed from others by a cheerful exterior. Peace-loving people who are distressed by quarrels. They can laugh at worries because they are aware of their unimportance. Helps transfer energy from lower centers to higher.

CENTAURY: Weak-willed; too easily influenced; willing servitors; submissive, timid. "We must earnestly learn to develop individuality according to the dictates of our own Soul." Positive: One who serves quietly and willingly, uninfluenced by others.

WALNUT: For people easily influenced by the strong opinions of others. The link-breaker. "Walnut is the Remedy of advancing stages, teething, puberty, change of life. For the big decisions made during life, such as change of religion, occupation or country."

HOLLY: Hatred, envy, jealousy, suspicion, anger. Active, intense types. "Holly protects us from everything that is not Universal Love."

For despondency or despair:

LARCH: Lack of confidence, anticipation of failure; inferiority complex; despondency. Positive Qualities: People who take the plunge into life; analytical and confident, sensitive.

PINE: Self-reproach, guilt, despondency. Blame themselves for everything that goes wrong. Of Pine, Willow, Rock Water and Larch, Dr. Bach said "(They need to realize that) one trace of condemnation against ourselves, or others, is a trace of condemnation against the Universal Creation of Love and restricts us and limits our power to allow Universal Love to flow through to others." These people will help others when needed, and persevere.

ELM: For those who are able and responsible, doing their life's work, but at times feel it is too much for them. Temporary faltering of self-confidence. Elm brings one back to earth. Helps materialize dearest hopes and wishes. Aligns centers.

SWEET CHESTNUT: Extreme mental anguish. For "The hopeless despair of those who feel they have reached the limit of their endurance." These are people of strong character. In the moment of anguish "the cry for help is heard and it is the moment when miracles are done."

STAR OF BETHLEHEM: For shock, after-effects of shock; refusal to be consoled. Restores balance. "The comforter and soother of pains and sorrows."

WILLOW: Resentment, bitterness, anger. Positive: Optimism and faith, accepting responsibility.

OAK: Despondency, despair, but unceasing effort. People who struggle on in the face of every difficulty. They never give up hope. "They are brave people, fighting against great difficulties without loss of hope or slackening of effort."

CRAB APPLE: Feel the need of cleansing of mind and body. Preoccupation with trivia. Restores us to our sense of proportion, singleness of purpose in creativity.

Over-care for the welfare of others:

CHICORY: Possessiveness, self-love, self-pity, perfectionism. "The cause of all our troubles is self and separateness, and this vanishes as soon as Love and the knowledge of the great Unit become part of our natures."

VERVAIN: Strain, stress, tension, over-enthusiasm. Tries to convert others. "It is the Remedy against over-effort. It teaches us that it is by *being* rather than doing that great things are accomplished."

VINE: Dominating, inflexible, ambitious, efficient, strong-willed. Positive: The wise, loving and understanding healer, leader or teacher who inspires others.

BEECH: Intolerant, critical, judgmental, lacking humility and compassion. Irritation with others comes out in rashes and allergies. "We need to be more tolerant, lenient and understanding of the different way each individual and all things are working toward their final perfection." Positive: Apply love wisely and wisdom lovingly.

ROCK WATER: Self-repression, self-denial, inflexibility. Hard masters on themselves. Positive: Reservoirs of energy. Emphasize the art of living. Love yourself.

APPENDIX C

Games

Dictionary Game

For four or more players. You'll need a dictionary, paper and pencils. One person (the starter) goes first and chooses a word from the dictionary whose meaning she or he doesn't think any other player knows. It can't be a word starting with a capital letter. The starter reads only the word and then writes down the dictionary definition in his or her own words. Each player writes a definition that seems right or invents one that's amusing. Then everyone passes in his or her definition to the starter, who reads all of them, not distinguishing between the dictionary definition and the rest (which means reading over them first in case someone's writing isn't clear). Everyone then guesses which is the "right" definition. Then the starter reads the dictionary definition. A player gets 10 points for writing the dictionary definition and 5 points if he or she guesses one someone else wrote. Play until you're tired of playing and add up the points . . . if anyone cares. In my family we don't often bother to keep score. We just do it for the laughs.

Analogy

For as many players as you want. One person (the starter) secretly picks a person in the room. If there aren't many of you, include someone whom everyone knows. Each player uses an analogy to get clues about who this person is. The object, obviously, is to name the person. The players ask, "If she or he were a bird, what kind of bird would she or he be?" "If she or he were a flower, instrument, cloud, car, etc. . . .?" The starter answers with the kind of bird, etc.— "She'd be a seagull or a pelican." As soon as you have a feeling who it might be, guess!

APPENDIX D: Reflexology Foot & Hand Charts

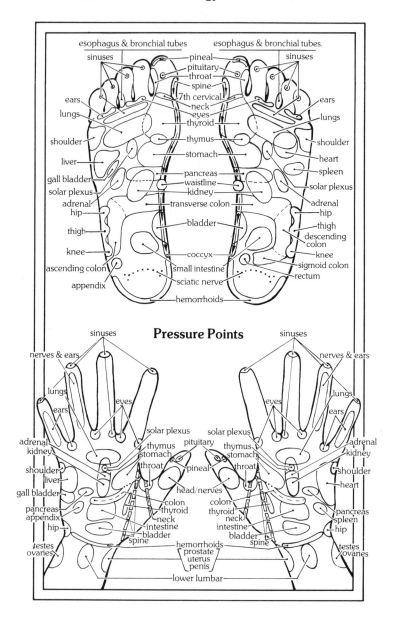

Reflexology Foot Charts

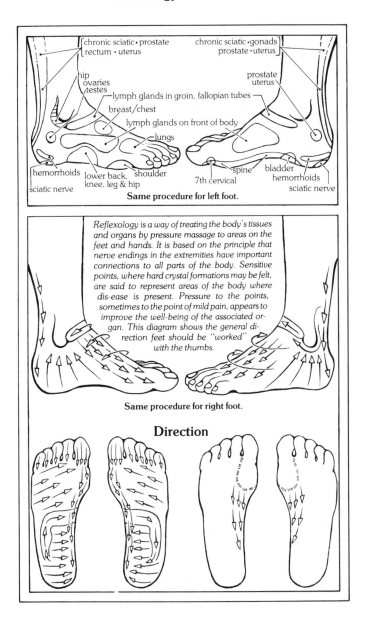

chronic sciatic • prostate
rectum • uterus

chronic sciatic • gonads
prostate • uterus

hip
ovaries
testes

prostate
uterus

lymph glands in groin, fallopian tubes

breast/chest

lymph glands on front of body

lungs

hemorrhoids

lower back,
knee, leg & hip

shoulder

sciatic nerve

spine

7th cervical

bladder
hemorrhoids

sciatic nerve

Same procedure for left foot.

Reflexology is a way of treating the body's tissues and organs by pressure massage to areas on the feet and hands. It is based on the principle that nerve endings in the extremities have important connections to all parts of the body. Sensitive points, where hard crystal formations may be felt, are said to represent areas of the body where dis-ease is present. Pressure to the points, sometimes to the point of mild pain, appears to improve the well-being of the associated organ. This diagram shows the general direction feet should be "worked" with the thumbs.

Same procedure for right foot.

Direction

-263-

APPENDIX E

Comparison of Right to Die Laws

	Arkansas ACT 879 March, 1977	California A.B. 3060 September, 1976
Title		Natural Death Act
Purpose	Permits an individual to "request or refuse in writing . . . procedures calculated to prolong his life."	To recognize the right of adult person to make a written directive instructing physician to withhold or withdraw life-sustaining procedures in event of terminal condition.
Who May Elect?	Any adult. Also permits a proxy to execute document on behalf of minor or incompetent.	Any adult person.
How to Elect	Voluntary execution of a document requiring two witnesses and notarization. For minors and incompetents, document can be executed by specified family members.	Voluntary execution of Directive to Physician, legally binding when executed 14 days after diagnosis of terminal condition; otherwise it is advisory.
Is Form Included?	No.	Yes.
Formalities of Execution	As with a will of property, two witnesses and notarization of document.	Directive requires 2 witnesses not related, nor entitled to estate nor in employ of physician. Must be made part of patient's medical record.
How Long is Document Effective?	In force unless revoked.	5 years.
When Does Document Become Controlling?	Law is imprecise except to state person's right to "die with dignity."	1) Certification of terminal condition by 2 physicians; 2) attending physician must determine validity of directive; 3) death must be "imminent" in judgment of physician.
Revocation Procedures Specified?	No.	Yes.
Is Document Binding on Physicians?	No penalty for non-compliance.	Yes. Unprofessional conduct for failure to comply unless arrangements made to transfer patients.
Are There Immunity Provisions?	Yes, for "person, hospital or other medical institution."	Yes, for physician, health facility and health professionals.
Penalties for Destruction, Concealment, Falsification Of Directive or Revocation	No.	Yes.

Idaho S.B. 1164 March, 1977	Kansas S.B. 99 April, 1979	Nevada A.B. 8 May, 1977
Natural Death Act		
To recognize right to execute written directive instructing physician to withhold or withdraw life-sustaining procedures when such a person is in a terminal condition.	To recognize an adult's right to make a written declaration instructing the physician to withhold or withdraw life-sustaining procedures in the event of a terminal condition.	To protect the terminal, comatose patient by means of an advance directive which is advisory only to physician.
Adult persons diagnosed as terminal.	Any adult person.	Any adult person.
Voluntary execution of a document which is legally binding if executed after diagnosis of a terminal condition.	Voluntary execution at any time of a written document directing the withholding or withdrawing of life-sustaining procedures in the event of a terminal illness.	Voluntary execution of "Directive to Physicians."
Yes.	Yes, but may include other specific directions.	Yes, but need only be followed "substantially."
Signed, written directive, two witnesses with same exclusions as California. Requires notarization.	Signed, written, witnessed directive, same witness exclusions as California. Permits signing by another on behalf of declarant, incapable of so doing, in his/her presence and under his/her direction.	Directive requires two witnesses, same exclusions as California. Must be made part of patient's record.
5 years.	In effect unless revoked.	In force unless revoked.
After determination by attending physician that death is imminent if patient is unable to communicate instructions.	Upon certification of terminal condition by two physicians.	Advisory only.
Yes.	Yes.	Yes.
No penalty for noncompliance.	Yes. Failure to comply or effect the transfer of a qualified patient constitutes unprofessional conduct.	No. Physician shall give weight to declaration but may consider other factors.
Yes, for physicians and health facilities.	Yes, for physician, health-care professionals, medical care facilities.	Yes, for physician, hospital, health professional.
No.	Yes.	Yes.

Comparison of Right to Die Laws (Cont'd)

	New Mexico S.B. 16 April, 1977	North Carolina S.B. 504 June, 1977
Title	Right to Die Act.	Right to a Natural Death; Brain Death.
Purpose	To allow an adult of sound mind to execute a document directing withholding of maintenance medical treatment when certified as terminal; also has provisions for terminally-ill minor.	To provide a procedure for the individual's right to a peaceful and natural death.
Who May Elect?	1) Adult of sound mind. 2) On behalf of a terminally-ill minor by specified family members with court certification.	Competent individual. No age provision specified. Also on behalf of terminal, comatose patients by specified family members.
How to Elect	Voluntary execution of document with same formalities as will. On behalf of minor by family member after certification of terminal condition by two physicians and requiring court certification of document.	Voluntary execution of an advisory document directing the withholding or discontinuance of extraordinary means.
Is Form Included?	No.	Yes, a suggested form to meet requirements of law: "Declaration of a Desire for a Natural Death."
Formalities of Execution	Requires two witnesses and notarization.	Signed declaration with 2 witnesses, same exclusions as California. Must be "Proved" before notary or clerk of court.
How Long is Document Effective?	In effect unless revoked.	Valid until revoked.
When Does Document Become Controlling?	After certification of terminal illness by two physicians.	Upon certification of terminal condition by 2 physicians.
Revocation Procedures Specified?	Yes.	Yes.
Is Document Binding on Physicians?	Yes, but no penalty for noncompliance.	No. Only advisory.
Are There Immunity Provisions?	Yes.	Yes.
Penalties for Destruction, Concealment, Falsification Of Directive or Revocation	Yes.	No.

Oregon S.B. 438 June, 1977	Texas S.B. 148 August, 1977	Washington H.B. 264 March, 1979
Act Relating to the Right to Die.	Natural Death Act	Natural Death Act
To allow an individual to execute or re-execute a directive directing the withholding or withdrawal of life-sustaining procedures should declarant become a qualified patient.	To establish a procedure for a person to provide in advance for the withdrawal or withholding of life-sustaining procedures in event of a terminal condition.	To allow adults to control decisions relating to their own medical care, including decision to have life-sustaining procedures withheld or withdrawn in event of terminal condition.
Adult of sound mind.	Any adult person	Any person at least 18 years old, of sound mind.
Directive must be signed 14 days after diagnosis and certification of terminal illness to be legally binding.	Voluntary execution of Directive to Physicians legally binding when executed after the diagnosis of a terminal condition; otherwise it is advisory.	Voluntary execution of advance directive directing the withholding or withdrawal of life-sustaining procedures in a terminal condition.
Yes.	Yes.	Yes, but may include other specific directions.
Directive requires 2 witnesses not related, nor entitled to estate nor in employ of physician. Directive must be placed in patient's medical record.	Directive requires 2 witnesses not related, nor entitled to estate nor in employ of physician. Must be made part of patient's medical record.	Signed declaration, requiring two witnesses with same exclusions as California. To be made part of patient's medical record.
Five years.	In force until revoked.	In force unless revoked.
When attending physician determines "death is imminent" and when life-prolonging procedures would only prolong dying. Physician need not determine validity of directive.	Upon diagnosis and certification of terminal condition by two physicians (one the attending). Physician must determine validity of directive.	Upon written verification of terminal condition by two physicians when life-sustaining procedures would only prolong "moment of death."
Yes.	Yes.	Yes.
No. Shall make "reasonable effort" to transfer patient.	Yes. Unprofessional conduct for failure to comply unless arrangements made to transfer patient.	No. Must make a "good faith effort" to transfer patient.
Yes.	Yes.	Yes. Physician, health personnel and facility.
Yes.	Yes	Yes.

APPENDIX F

Some Holistic Healing Techniques and Terms

Acupressure: A finger pressure technique that breaks through energy flow blockages by releasing muscular tension. Acupressure uses the same system of points and meridians as acupuncture, but instead of placing needles through the skin, it works by manual pressure on tension blocks under the skin surface. *

Acupuncture: Therapy form developed in China which understands health and disease in terms of the balance or imbalance of energy flows (chi) within the body. These flows of energy are either stimulated or dispersed by inserting needles into specific points on the skin, by applying heat, by pressure, by massage, or by a combination of these. The system includes basic holistic principles and practices including the five-elements theory, the cyclical laws of nature, dietary considerations, etc. *

Affirmations: Positive statements about oneself or one's situation, often used in creative visualization to focus one's attention and will on a desired result. Affirmations may be precisely specific or quite general. *

Aikido: In its purely practical application, an art of self-defense. However, aikido is more than a physical art. Its techniques are interwoven with elements of philosophy, psychology, and dynamics. It is a way of being that unites life energy (ki) into harmony with one's environment. *

Allopathy: Conventional systemic and symptomatic medicine as known and practiced by most physicians today. Deals generally with treatment and prevention of physical disease rather than with maintenance and improvement of health. *

Art therapy: Free artistic expression used for diagnostic and therapeutic purposes, or as an objective means of following the progress of a particular therapy. *

Astrology: The science and art of astrology tells us precisely where the planets are at a given time and interprets the meaning of changing relationships between the planets. There is a meaningful correspondence, a 'synchronicity', between the outer worlds and earth which can facilitate understanding the patterns and possibilities in our everyday lives. A horoscope is a map of the positions of all the planets at the moment of birth, believed to be a pattern basic to understanding the personality, abilities and challenges of the individual.

Aura balancing: Process of realigning electromagnetic energy (the aura) to bring greater harmony among body, feelings, mind and soul. Based on view that human beings are inherently loving and have an inner reality more potent than any challenges.

Biofeedback: Technique by which one can learn conscious control of biological processes (especially those once thought to be involuntary by Western science) by means of subliminal information about the process that is obtained by electrical measuring instruments and fed back to the individual. *

Chiropractic: Based on theory that misalignment of vertebrae produces blockages of nerve function which causes unlimited symptoms and system malfunctions that can be cured by physical adjustments to the spine.

Color therapy: Use of the light waves or energy of particular colors for healing purposes.

Do-in: A technique for giving acupressure to oneself. It uses knowledge of the effects of specific points to obtain temporary relief. *

Dream Work: Techniques of using dreams as a means of bringing unconscious feelings, thoughts and patterns to conscious awareness.

Encounter: Approach to personality integration that encourages participants to be open and honest in a group setting, often eliciting emotions that lead to confrontation.

Feldenkrais exercises: Simple and often effective exercises developed by Moshe Feldenkrais to use body energy more naturally and efficiently to retrain the brain's habitual response patterns.

Gestalt therapy: Theory and approach to personality integration originally developed by Fritz and Laura Perls that uses immediate excitement and awareness to develop personal responsibility.

Guided fantasy: Techniques where structured fantasy (stories, characters, situations) is used for the study or activiation of subpersonalities, or personal archetypes, involving their attitudes toward a current problem or situation, and to obtain access to other contents of the unconscious mind. *

Herbs: Plants used for their medicinal qualities.

Homeopathy: A healing system based on the principle that "like cures like." Homeopathic physicians believe that a remedy has the potential to cure a disease if it produces symptoms (similar to those of the disease) in a healthy organism. Another basic premise of homeopathy is that there are no diseases as such, only 'diseased individuals.' *

Iridology: Diagnosis of health from markings that appear in close examination of the eye.

Martial arts: Oriental disciplines evolved from the path of the Warrior, which properly used can lead to spiritual and physical integration, *e.g.,* Aikido, Karate, Kung Fu, T'ai Chi. *

Massage: A healing art that uses physical touch and manipulation to relax the body, balance and free energy, and soothe the mind and feelings.

Meditation: Quiet, deep level awareness. Meditation is not a single practice, and thus not easily defined. It encompasses diverse methods such as formal sitting (as in *zazen* or Vipassana), in which the body is held immobile and the attention controlled; expressive practices (such as Siddha Yoga, the Latihan, or the chaotic meditation of Rajneesh), in which the body is set free and anything can happen; and even the practice of going about one's daily round of activities mindfully (as in Mahamudra, Shiken Taza, or Gurdjieff's "self-remembering"). *

Movement therapy: The use of dance and other forms of directed physical movement for healing effects. *

Music therapy: Certain kinds of music employed to achieve specific health restoring and promoting goals, including heightened awareness and acceptance of all parts of the self.

Neoreichian therapy: A type of breathing activity developed from the work of Wilhelm Reich to release emotional patterns locked in the body. Yelling, crying, laughing, pounding, kicking, etc., are often used as part of the technique.

Polarity therapy: A science and practice of balancing the life energy in the human body. Objectives are to discover the anatomical relationship and function of the vital energy circuits and fields by which the body was built and continues to function, as "plus and minus" energy polarities, and to balance them by scientific skill rather than by force of mechanics. This is done through gentle hand contact, loving thought and attitude, exercise, and diet. *

Postural integration: A form of deep connective tissue manipulation. Greater emphasis on the entire being, physical and emotional, distinguishes it from Rolfing. P.I. sessions often include Reichian breathing work and polarity manipulations. *

Psychosynthesis: An inclusive approach to growth developed by Roberto Assagioli that focuses on expressing the will of the Higher Self.

Psychic healing: Healing energy from universal sources is transmitted consciously by the practitioner (or the afflicted person) mentally, by laying on hands or by "absent healing" (from a distance).

Rebirthing: Practitioners guide a person to relive the birth process—thereby releasing the trauma of birth.

Reflexology: Foot zone therapy. Pressure and massage primarily to the toes and soles of the feet are used to stimulate nerve endings in the feet to promote healing in specific areas of the body.

Rolfing: A technique of deep manipulation of the musculo-skeletal system to bring its major segments—head, shoulders, thorax, and legs—toward a vertical alignment. The technique often stimulates painful areas which are thought to contain 'blockages' brought on by a person's past experiences and habits. Alignment relieves these patterns and allows the person to develop new ones. Developed by Ida P. Rolf.*

Shiatsu: A traditional form of Japanese finger-pressure massage used as a preventive health measure. Contact is made by slow, deep penetration of key points along acupuncture meridians.

T'ai chi ch'uan: Traditional series of movements that are intended to unite consciousness of body and mind. It is a form of spiritual and physical exercise and probably originated with the early Taoists.*

Tarot: An ancient set of 78 picture images representing fundamental human archetypal energy patterns. They have been found useful in a system in which the practitioner uses conscious and unconscious faculties to interpret the relationship of the Tarot symbols to an individual's life and unconscious knowing.

Visualization: Creative means for using imagination to positively transform any life situation. Visualization includes processes of forming images and thoughts in the mind, and then transmitting them to the body as signals or commands.*

Yoga: (Sanskrit—"to yoke, join, fasten or harness.") Meditative work to concentrate and focus the mind in order to obtain union with universal spirit. Techniques and underlying philosophy which help to bring about a natural balance of body and mind in which the state of health can manifest itself. Yoga is an applied science of the mind and body stemming from the Indian philosophical system of Samkhva.*

*Adapted from *The Holistic Health Handbook*, compiled by Berkeley Holistic Health Center, And/Or Press, 1978.

APPENDIX G

Directive to Physicians
(Sample from Texas)

Directive made this _____ day of _____ (month, year).

I _____, being of sound mind, willfully and voluntarily make known my desire that my life shall not be artificially prolonged under the circumstances set forth below, and do hereby declare:

1. If at any time I should have an incurable condition caused by injury, disease, or illness certified to be a terminal condition by two physicians, and where the application of life-sustaining procedures would serve only to artificially prolong the moment of my death and where my attending physician determines that my death is imminent whether or not life-sustaining procedures are utilized, I direct that such procedures be withheld or withdrawn, and that I be permitted to die naturally.

2. In the absence of my ability to give directions regarding the use of such life-sustaining procedures, it is my intention that this directive shall be honored by my family and physicians as the final expression of my legal right to refuse medical or surgical treatment and accept the consequences from such refusal.

3. If I have been diagnosed as pregnant and that diagnosis is known to my physician, this directive shall have no force or effect during the course of my pregnancy.

4. I have been diagnosed and notified as having a terminal condition by _____ _____, M.D., whose address is _____ and whose telephone number is _____. I understand that if I have not filled in the physician's name and address, it shall be presumed that I did not have a terminal condition when I made out this directive.

5. This directive shall be in effect until it is revoked.

6. I understand the full import of this directive and I am emotionally and mentally competent to make this directive.

7. I understand that I may revoke this directive at any time.

Signed _____
City, County, and State Residence _____

The declarant has been personally known to me and I believe him or her to be of sound mind. I am not related to the declarant by blood or marriage, nor would I be entitled to any portion of the declarant's estate on his decease, nor am I the attending physician of declarant or an employee of the attending physician or a health facility in which declarant is a patient, or a patient in the health care facility in which the declarant is a patient, or any person who has a claim against any portion of the estate of the declarant upon his decease.

Witness _____
Witness _____

Before me, the undersigned authority, on this day personally appeared _____ _____, _____, and _____, known to me to be the declarant and witnesses whose names are subscribed to the foregoing instrument in their respective capacities, and, all of said persons being by me duly sworn, the declarant, _____, declared to me and to the said witnesses in my presence that said instrument is his Directive to Physicians, and that he had willingly and voluntarily made and executed it as his free act and deed for the purposes therein expressed.

Declarant _____

Witness _____

Witness _____

Subscribed and acknowledged before me by the said Declarant, _____
_____, and by the said witnesses, _____and
_____, on this _____ day of _____, 19_____.

_____
Notary Public in and for _____ County.

APPENDIX H

References

About Dying. A Scriptographic Booklet, Channing L. Bete Co., New Haven CT, 1978.

Ars Moriendi (Dying Arts). Walter J. Johnson edition. (One of the world's first do-it-yourself books, it taught the art of dying. Original was published in Florence in 1488. A modern English edition was published by Arno Press, New York, 1977.)

Bach, Marcus, *I Monty.* Island Heritage, Ltd., Norfolk Island, Australia, 1977. (Available from Association for Research and Enlightenment, P.O. Box 595, Virginia Beach, VA 23451.)

Berkeley Holistic Health Center, *The Holistic Health Handbook.* And/Or Press, Berkeley, CA, 1978.

Blake, William, *Notebook.* Geoffrey Keynes, ed., Cooper Square, Totowa, NJ, 1971.

Boone J. Allen, *Kinship with All Life.* Harper and Row, New York, 1976.

The Brain Mind Bulletin (newsletter). Marilyn Ferguson, ed., Interface Press, P.O. Box 42211, Los Angeles, CA 90042.

Bricklin, Mark, *The Practical Encyclopedia of Natural Healing.* Rodale Press, Emmaus, PA, 1976.

Caxton, William, (translator), *Art and Craft to Knowe Ye Well to Dye.* William Caxton, Westminster, England, 1490. (Written in the fifteenth century, this book included instructions for everything from the art of blowing your nose to weeping well.)

The Center for Attitudinal Healing
A Course in Miracles. Celestial Arts, Millbrae, CA, 1979.
There's a Rainbow Behind Every Dark Cloud. (Written by the children at the center.)

Clark, Linda, *Color Therapy.* Devin-Aclair, Old Greenwich, CT, 1975.

Coughlin, George G., *Law for the Layman.* Harper and Row, New York, 1975.

Cousins, Norman, *Anatomy of an Illness as Perceived by the Patient: Reflections on Healing and Regeneration.* W. W. Norton and Co., New York, 1979.

Ferguson, Marilyn, *The Aquarian Conspiracy.* J.P. Tarcher, Publisher, Los Angeles, CA, 1979.

Fortune, Dion, *Through the Gates of Death.* Samuel Weiser, York Beach, ME, 1968.

Frankl, Victor, *Man's Search for Meaning: An Introduction to Logotherapy.* Beacon Press, Boston, MA, 1959. (Victor Frankl is a psychiatrist who survived Auschwitz and Dachau. After his experiences there he would state, "The salvation of man is through love and in love.")

Fynn, *Mister God, This is Anna.* Ballantine Books, New York, 1974. (For older children and adults—a book I love that deals with a spiritual understanding of life and death.)

Gibran, Kahlil, *The Prophet.* Alfred A. Knopf, New York, 1967.

Gordon, James S., M.D., *Holistic Medicine: Introduction and Overview.* Published by the U.S. Government and available through the Institute of Noetic Sciences, 600 Stockton Street, San Francisco, CA 94108.

The Gospel According to Thomas. (A. Guillaumont *et al.,* translators of the apocryphal Coptic text.) Harper and Row, New York, 1957.

Gray, V. Ruth, *Dealing with Death and Dying, Some Physiological Needs.* Nursing 77 Books, Nursing Skill Book Service, Jenkintown, PA, 1976.

Grof, Stanislav, and Joan Halifax, *The Human Encounter with Death.* E. P. Dutton, New York, 1978.

The Hanuman Foundation Dying Project Newsletter. (The Hanuman Foundation was founded by Ram Dass, an American spiritual teacher. The Dying Project, directed by Stephen Levine, publishes this newsletter on death and dying. Write P.O. Box 2228, Taos, NM 87571.)

Heline, Corinne, "Color and Music in the New Age," *New Age*, 1964.

Huxley, Laura, *This Timeless Moment.* Celestial Arts, Millbrae, CA, 1975. (Describes the death of Aldous Huxley, an innovative adventurer in the human mind. Huxley used LSD in his last days in order to experience his death as fully as possible.)

Illich, Ivan, *Medical Nemesis.* Pantheon, New York, 1976. (A scholarly and intriguing history of attitudes and practices about death.)

Internal Revenue Service
 A Guide to Federal Estate and Gift Taxation (No. 448)
 Tax Information for Survivors (No. 559)

Jampolsky, Gerald, *Love is Letting Go of Fear.* Celestial Arts, Millbrae, CA, 1979. (A useful guide for transforming one's life, including the fear and pain.)

Khan, Hazrat Inayat, *The Purpose of Life.* The Rainbow Bridge Bookstore, San Francisco, 1973.

Kübler-Ross, Dr. Elisabeth
 Death, the Final State of Growth. Prentice-Hall, Englewood Cliffs, NJ, 1975.
 Questions and Answers on Death and Dying. Prentice-Hall, Englewood Cliffs, NJ, 1978.
 To Live Until We Say Goodbye. Prentice-Hall, Englewood Cliffs, NJ, 1978.
 On Death and Dying. MacMillan, New York, 1980.
 Living With Death and Dying. MacMillan, New York, 1981.
 A Letter to a Child with Cancer. (The "Dougy Letter," a beautiful explanation of life and death that children can understand, available from Shanti Nilaya.)
 "Life, Death and Life after Death." (cassette tape)
 "Dr. Kübler-Ross Talks to High School Students." (cassette tape)
  (Tapes and "Dougy Letter" are available from Shanti Nilaya, P.O. Box 2396, Escondido, CA 92095.)

Lack, Sylvia A., *Psychosocial Care of the Dying Patient.* Charles Garfield (ed.), McGraw Hill, New York, 1978. (Originally a paper given before the First National Training Conference for Physicians on Psychosocial Care of the Dying Patient, April 29, 1976. Sylvia A. Lack is a national hospice organizer.)

LeShan, Eda, *Learning to Say Goodbye.* Macmillan, New York 1976. (Also available as an Avon paperback. A loving, sensitive book an older child age 9-10 can read to him or herself, or which a remaining parent or child can benefit from sharing.)

Levine, Stephen, *The Gradual Awakening.* Doubleday, New York, 1979.

Lipnack, Jessica (ed.), "Dying: New Age Readers Respond," *New Age* magazine, March, 1978.

Lopez, Barry (ed.), "The American Indian Mind," *Omni* magazine. Sept.-Oct. 1978. (Section on "Knowing how to die," p. 113.)

Maclean, Dorothy, *To Hear the Angels Sing.* Findhorn Publications, Moray, Scotland, 1980. (A teenager or an adult might feel less alone after reading this.)

Make Today Count (newsletter). 1137 Colusa Ave., Berkeley, CA 74707. (Started by a courageous cancer patient who died recently, this organization publishes a free newsletter and holds frequent meetings for sharing the challenges of a life-threatening disease.)

Marback, Ethel, *The Cabbage Moth and the Shamrock.* Star and Elephant Books, Green Tiger Press, La Jolla, CA, 1978.

Miriam, Satya, *Healing Is Transformation: The Opening of the Rose.* Baraka Books, New York, 1978.

Moody, Raymond, M.D.
   Life After Life. Stackpole Books, Harrisburg, PA, 1976. (Experiences recorded by the author, including repeated confirmations there will be beautiful light, love and loving people to meet the dying person.)
   Reflections on Life After Life. Bantam Books, New York, 1977.

Morgan, Ernest. *A Manual of Death Education and Simple Burial.* Celo Press, Route 5, Burnsville, NC 17814, 1977. (Available for $2, postpaid. Also available through memorial societies.)

Muggeridge, Malcolm. *Something Beautiful for God.* Doubleday, New York, 1977. (A book about Mother Theresa.)

Muir, John. *The Velvet Monkey Wrench.* John Muir Publications, Santa Fe, NM, 1973.

Neihardt, John G., *Black Elk Speaks.* University of Nebraska Press, Lincoln, NB, 1961.

Osis, Dr. Karlis and Erlendur Haraldsson, "Deathbed Observations by Physicians and Nurses: A Cross-Cultural Survey," in *The Journal for the American Society of Psychical Research,* and published as *Parapsychological Monograph No. 3,* Parapsychology Foundation, 1961.

Perry, Whitall N., *A Treasury of Traditional Wisdom.* Simon and Schuster, New York, 1971. (Thoughts of St. Augustine, Black Elk, and others are included in this book.)

Rajneesh Foundation Newletter
   "Here Comes a Fresh Breeze of God," *Rajneesh Foundation Newsletter,* Volume III, No. 18, September 16, 1977.

Rawlings, Maurice, M.D., *Beyond Death's Door.* Nelson, Nashville, TN, 1978.

Seiver, George, *The Man and His Mind.* Harper and Row, New York, 1976.

Shepard, Martin, *Someone You Love is Dying: A Guide for Helping and Coping.* Harmony Books, Crown Publishers, Inc., New York, 1975.

Stern, Phillip, *Lawyers on Trial,* Times Books, New York, 1980.

Waterman, Robert, *Self Forgiveness: An Act of Life.* Southwestern College of Life Sciences, Alamogordo, NM, 1976.

White Eagle, *The Quiet Mind.* Fletcher and Son, Ltd., Norwich, England, 1972. (This is a beautiful little book from England I've used for years to help me relax and sleep well. It's available through some metaphysical bookstores and Shanti Nilaya.)

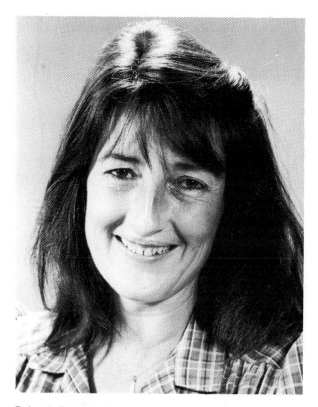

Deborah Duda was born in Ohio and lived in many parts of the world as a daughter of a military family. She was a foreign service officer and a fashion designer, and for the past nine years has been actively involved with helping people accept dying as a natural part of life. She lives on Kauai, Hawaii.

If you would like another copy or copies of *Coming Home* by Deborah Duda, please fill out the form below and sent it and your check or money order to:

John Muir Publications
P.O. Box 613
Santa Fe, NM 87504

Ship to: _____

    Address _____

        City _____ State _____ Zip _____

_____

Please send _____ copies of *Coming Home* @ $8.95 each.   Total _____

                                 Postage _____1.50___

Add 44¢ per copy for tax if you live in
           Sunny New Mexico   Total _____

                     Total Enclosed _____